U R Here
Always

A Novel

By Joseph Belan

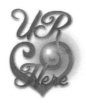

DEDICATION

This book is dedicated to my beautiful and courageous
wife, Sharon.

It is also dedicated to all of the families that have had to
suffer from the ravages of Ovarian Cancer,
as well as to those skilled heath care professionals from
Great Lakes Hospice.

May they all be blessed.

***

Published by: JB Publishing LLC
Copyrighted by: Joseph Belan, 2013.
All Rights Reserved.

For information, contact the publisher:

JB Publishing LLC
5227 MIll Sreet
Erie, PA 16509

Library of Congress Number (ISBN):
978-09889554-1-7

© Joscph Belan

U R Here Always:
A novel based on a true story of a man's love in sickness and in health. Cancer took Sharon from Joe's life, nothing can take Sharon from Joe's heart.

Second Edition - $19.95 + $6.00 S&H
Printed in the United States of America

Cover and logo designed by RUKE (www.ruke.com)

ACKNOWLEDGMENTS

The author would like to acknowledge the following people: Kim Burney, Daniel Ruke, Maureen McBride, Amy Bovaird, Frank Strumila, Glenn, Patty, Ellen Miller, Steven and Michael Skelly, Patricia Tassone, Hallie Estepp, Heather Pisciotti, and Jason Belan.

Thank you all.

INTRODUCTION

Join me on an inspiring journey: celebrate with me the last fifteen years of Sharon Belan's life. You may not know her, but you can know her story. Experience her dreams, watch her travel through lands that she makes magical, despite grim odds. Watch her meet her life and its challenges with childlike awe.

You will experience a recovery from physical and emotional pain and disappointment as if it was your wife or loved one. You will feel the joy and faith that Sharon felt as she filled the final years of her life, changing despair into hope, shining light into everyone's life. Look to the light. Always.

Chapter 1
THE DIAGNOSIS

With a score of four under par after only eight holes, this round was the best I'd ever golfed and not just since retirement. On the ninth hole I was in a position to birdie or at least par. I addressed the ball for my second shot on the long par five, thinking I could be on the green in two shots with the possibility of an eagle, at six strokes under par, a score that up till now had been impossible for me to achieve.

Focus, Joe, focus.

I saw a stark raving lunatic speed across the fairway shouting and waving his arms. Even a novice knew never to make noise or distract a golfer when he addressed his ball. *Golfing 101.*

This fool better have a damn good explanation.

I stepped away from my ball and gestured with a furious what-the-hell-are-you-thinking motion. I was ready to light into the jerk when I recognized Rush Trace, the owner of the course.

I froze, golf club-in-hand. He would never interrupt my swing without a helluva good reason.

My heart beat in a staccato rhythm as his golf cart stopped within inches of me. Rush waved a cell phone at me. "Call home."

I searched his face for a sign that this call merited disrupting a once-in-a-lifetime round of golf. Concern pulled his features taught on his face but then he always wore that expression. "Take your time. Return the phone whenever you can."

My world slowed to a crawl. I watched him drive away until he disappeared from view. Then I looked down at the phone. It felt heavy in my hand. What did I need to do?

I simply stared for a moment. Then his words penetrated my befuddled brain: *phone home.*

Shoving my club into the bag, I shot into action. As fast as I could, I punched in the numbers to reach Sharon, my wife of five years. *Was she okay?* I willed the electronic impulse to speed through space faster than physics allowed. On a typical day, she answered the phone on the third or fourth ring. But not today. She answered it even before the first ring finished. She must have been sitting there with her cell phone in hand, ready to answer at the first sign of my callback.

Panic struck my heart—that same gut fear I had when my principal called me away from my classroom to tell me that my daughter had been killed in a car accident.

The physical. She'd had an exam scheduled earlier with Dr. Peter Sturm, our family doctor. *Oh God. They found something.*

"Shar. Are you okay?"

"Joe. Thank God it's you." She released an audible sigh. "The doctor wants me to go to the emergency room at St. Vincent's and check in. Please come home. I'll get my stuff ready, and wait for you." She sounded breathless.

"What happened? What did they find?"

"I don't know. Just *hurry*."

"I'm on my way." I felt the color drain from my face. Old guy that I was, I threw my 6'6" torso into gear, tore past my now abandoned ball, tossed my clubs into the cart and rushed to the pro shop, throwing the cell phone on the counter. I don't even remember getting into my Ford Explorer. I peeled out of the parking lot, soon exceeding the forty-mile speed limit by fifty-five miles per hour and took "Dead-Man's Curve" on Route 97 at eighty. I cut down a fifteen-to-twenty minute drive to five minutes going home. It's a wonder I made it alive.

She was waiting in a T-shirt and blue jeans, seated on the front porch, one hand on a small overnight bag and the other on her purse. She looked composed, as usual, her small frame perched forward on the edge of the chair, her face tilted toward the sun. I could envision the smattering of freckles on the creamy-white skin she complained never tanned. Seeing her in such a normal state—as if nothing had happened -- made me pause at the wheel, hungering for moments I'd taken for granted just this morning.

When I parked the car, she jumped up. Relief settled on her face when she saw me. I took her in my arms, as much to comfort myself as to give reassurance. I brushed her soft hair with a kiss and pushed her forward. "Let's go."

"Okay, ready."

I circled around to open the car door for her. *Damn bum knee!* It gave out on me, slowing me down just enough that she beat me to the door, fumbling with the handle.

Seated, she pulled the seatbelt around herself and snapped it into place with trembling fingers.

"What did the doctor say?" I backed out of the driveway. "Did he give you any clue at all as to what's wrong?"

She shook her head. "Just said I needed to get there ASAP. I'm as in-the-dark as you, Joe."

Oh God. Not good. "How could he leave you *hanging* like that?"

"…something about my lungs."

"Your *lungs?* You haven't been sick, have you? What's that all about?"

She shrugged. "I don't know. Calm down. If you drive like a fool, neither of us will make it to the hospital." Although, she tried to sound matter-of-a-fact, she must have been reeling inside. But she knew I loathed hospitals. They always turned out to be the last place I saw my loved ones alive.

The faster we got there, the sooner we'd know what was wrong. I stepped on the gas.

"Dear Lord, get us there in one piece." She gripped my hand, now on the gearshift. "It'll be okay, Joe." Knowing my emotional state, she tried to protect me. We did that a lot for each other.

"Right. First things first. Let's get you there."

At the emergency room, they took Sharon in and admitted her. That afternoon, they set her up to receive some tests, which continued throughout the next day.

Finally, the doctor came to the room. He sat down beside her. "I'm afraid I have some bad news for you, Sharon." She gave him a concerned glance as he continued. "You have a tumor on your ovary. It's large enough that it's pushing against your lungs and creating a lot of fluid. That's why we're draining it." Dr. Sturm pointed to a tube.

Sharon turned to me and gripped my arm. Her face paled. The doctor let the words sink in as our minds raced to the possibilities. In shock, I stroked her arm as she spoke. "Is this tumor can—"

"Cancerous?" His voice turned softer with compassion as he met the fear in Sharon's eyes. "Well, we don't know for sure. We do know that you have sixteen of the twenty-one symptoms, none of which would be alarming on their own. But together, they could add up to something more serious."

As that day ended, we were thrown into the biggest emotional battle we ever faced together. We learned what Dr. Sturm suspected: Sharon not only had ovarian cancer, but she was in the latter stages of it.

When you're as old as I am, having survived not one but two bad marriages, and you *finally* find the woman you've waited your entire life for, why is it that life kicks you in the gut like this? Damn it all to hell! No hospital is going to take Sharon down. We're going to beat this thing.

The hospital staff allowed me to stay overnight. As we lay in her bed, I whispered, "Don't worry. Remember, I have connections. That's one benefit from surviving cancer, huh? I'm going to call my oncologist tomorrow. He can put us in touch with the best ovarian specialist there is." I squeezed her hand.

"Can you find his number? It must be at home..." She leaned her head on my shoulder.

"I'll get it. I know exactly where it is." *You never lose those contacts.* Diagnosed with prostate cancer the same year we married, I followed the doctor's orders to a T. Yes, it did shake us up. But optimism prevailed. My oncologist had been terrific. If anyone could help us, it was he.

We spent half a day consulting with Dr. Joel Newton. "Look Doc, I don't care about money. I can liquidate my assets. Find me the best cancer specialist in the world."

Those were his marching orders. I hoped he could pull through for me. That he took time out of his busy schedule to look at all reassured me that he could do it. I felt the same trust I did when he cared for me four years earlier.

The call finally came. "Joe, here's the deal. I'm afraid to say it but the best doctor has moved out of UPMC. I've secured the second best doctor for you, and he's in residence right here at Magee. How about that? His name is Dr. Gene Clemente. He has a ninety-eight percent success rate in saving his cancer patients."

"Really? Man, I don't know how to thank you for the time you spent on our behalf." Words seemed inadequate. Dr. Newton had always extended himself, serving as much as a confidant as a doctor. I knew I'd never forget the way he put himself out to hook us up with this specialist.

Sharon sat up when I arrived at her bedside. When I

told her we'd found a superb doctor, she sank back into her pillow and smiled as if she knew all along we would.

"What's his name again?"

I looked through my sheath of papers from the call. "Dr. Clemente, I believe."

She lifted her hands and looked up. "Thank you, God," she mouthed. "Clemente? *Clemente*...I know that word from somewhere. Maybe it's Spanish. Yes! Hon, guess what? That's Spanish for *merciful*". Tears filled her eyes. "This is a really good sign."

I blinked in surprise. "You're quick. How do you know these things?" Something clicked in my brain just then. "You know what else? The Pittsburgh Pirates have a player named Clemente."

I sat down on the edge of her bed and smoothed the sheets before taking her hands and warming them between my own larger ones. "Of course it's a good sign." I kissed each of her fingers, marveling at how upbeat she seemed in spite of the circles under her eyes. "The best thing—they can take you right away, early in the morning, in fact. He's right at UPMC Magee Women's Hospital in Pittsburgh."

"Your neck of the woods," she said softly.

Chapter 2
MAGEE WOMEN'S HOSPITAL

The next morning, a technician strapped Sharon onto a gurney facing backward in the ambulance while I squeezed her hand.

"Sorry sir, we're still draining the fluid from her lungs, and we need the space for the apparatus," the technician said, sizing up my bulk. "You understand it's in your wife's best interest, don't you? We'll take good care of her."

She looked terrified, and I was trying to be the strong reassuring husband. *How can I do that when I can't even ride in the ambulance with her? Dammit!*

For the next two and a half hours, I followed the ambulance from St. Vincent's Hospital in Erie to Magee. I imagined Sharon looking out the rear window trying to find my car among the many on the road. She hated riding backward like this. She complained the motion sickness made her nauseous. Maybe the drugs and painkillers reduced a lot of her anxiety. At least I hoped that was the case. I wondered if she could see my face. Probably not, but I tried to smile and wave once in awhile, just in case.

I was smoking—and feeling guilty with every puff I took. The smoke curled up and around the steering wheel, then hung in the air and settled onto my clothing. *Uh-oh, she'll smell it!* I unrolled the window and waved it out, hoping she couldn't see me from where she lay in the ambulance. Hadn't she just said last week to one of our friends, 'I finally broke him of that nasty habit'? *Look at how easily you caved.* I flicked some ash out the window and recalled her pale face in the ambulance. Even at five car lengths away, I felt her frightened heart beating.

"Hang in there, babe. Everything's going to be all right," I said out loud. *Lord, we need you here. If anything bad happens, then let it happen to me.*

Dr. Sturm had said, "We need to get the ovarian cancer before it metastasizes and becomes inoperable." These words went round and round in my brain, circling like vultures, ready to devour any sense of comfort I felt, even knowing Dr. Clemente would be doing the surgery. Dr. Sturm had warned us to act fast.

In the hospital room at Magee, a pleasant young nurse entered the room. "Here's a menu. Choose whatever you want," she said kindly. Sharon selected a nice breakfast of scrambled eggs, bacon, coffee, and whole-wheat toast. About an hour after the nurse left with her order, another nurse arrived carrying the news that she would be operated on soon.

"Eat nothing." The second nurse marched out of the room without answering a single one of my questions.

We hadn't even spoken to Dr. Clemente yet. How

could we be scheduled for surgery when we didn't even know what it involved?

"Ohhhh." Sharon gave me her half-scared, half-starved look.

Like an enraged bear, I set my jaw forward prepared to intimidate. I hustled after the nurse, throwing questions at her back. "Can she have juice? No? What about coffee? Can she at least have some water? Anything at all? And what does 'soon' mean?"

The nurse didn't even slow down. As she disappeared into a windowless room, she repeated over her shoulder, "Soon means soon, and nothing by mouth."

Upon returning back to the room, I saw that the hopeful look on Sharon's face had vanished. I repeated the nurse's mandate.

"That's all right. You tried." She patted my hand.

Terrific. So I 'tried.' Fat lot of good I did. I could lobby in defense of a thousand striking teachers and get my own

way, but throw me in a hospital to fight for my wife, and

watch me strike out... I guess that nurse showed me.

Another hour passed. We talked on and off about everything except the pending operation.

Suddenly, the hospital door swung open. Dr. Clemente came bouncing in, overflowing with confidence, exuberance, and joy, as if he were going to slay the great ovarian cancer dragon and save the kingdom. We both fell in love with him because we felt he was 'that' good. Three of his minions followed him closely. They were more than interns. They were future ovarian cancer surgeon gods.

"Good morning—it's still morning, isn't it? I'm Dr. Clemente and this is my staff." He looked at her chart and said, "Aha! Nice to meet you, Sharon ... Belan, is it? It's unfortunate to meet under these circumstances, but that will soon be remedied, now won't it?" He proceeded to make small talk while probing her abdomen, kidneys, diaphragm and breasts. We learned that she would have another battery of blood tests, an x-ray and either an MRI or C-T scan.

Following that, she would be returned to the room to be prepped for surgery. We both knew what *that* meant. They were going to shave her. "Hey, I don't mind taking on that chore if you need a hand," I said, tongue-in-cheek. Shar gave me one of her 'looks.'

"Aw, Shar, why not? I don't need any specialized training for that job." Even this didn't get a rise or smile out of her. They were already explaining the other surgery procedures—they would stick needles into her hands and forearm to administer fluids and anesthetics. She grimaced.

How Sharon hated the sight of blood and the thought of sharp metal instruments being plunged into her body. Those things made her nauseous and light-headed. She tapped me on the wrist and I bent over to hear her better. "I detest the thought of being a pincushion," she whispered.

"I know, sweetheart. I know." My voice caught in my throat. The knight-in-shining-armor in me wanted to take this all away, but I couldn't and it was killing me.

After Clemente bounced merrily out of the room, we tried to support each other. "Remember, this is all good." I consoled.

"God is going to turn this whole cancer thing around starting today," she responded, making a motion as if she were changing a picture frame around. We continued with brave words, but we were actually clueless about what was about to happen.

When the kitchen server showed up with Sharon's breakfast, we stared at each other wondering which nurse had erred. We didn't have to wonder long. Immediately following the breakfast server came the mean nurse who dashed Sharon's breakfast hopes by snatching the tray and quickly marching away.

"There you go. God *does* have a sense of humor," I whispered tenderly with a fake growl as I imitated the mean nurse grabbing the tray and exiting.

About four o'clock, they took my wife away to administer all the tests. Around six, she returned to the room only to be assailed by a host of nurses armed with trays full of phlebotomy and anesthetic instruments. "Ahhh, it's the blood collectors," Sharon said in an attempt at dark humor. She didn't carry it off very well as she shrank back from the dreaded instruments and had to be coaxed into making a fist. They shooed me out until the nurses finished the prepping.

Shortly before seven, they let me back in the room. A small, rounded woman with short brown hair looking to be in her early forties popped in and sat down beside Sharon. "I'm Lisa Stall, a member of Dr. Clemente's team," she said, her voice warm and encouraging. "I know it's a scary time for you. Remember when you go into that operation, we need all your positive thoughts. You are a woman on a mission. Your mission is to get rid of these cancer cells, understand? And Dr. Clemente is the man to get it done."

That talk seemed to bolster my wife's morale. She sat up straighter and smiled.

After a long day of waiting for things to happen, we found ourselves in a flurry of activity when two aides rolled in a bed to transport Sharon to the operating room.

In the silence, Lisa Stall's words came to mind. *A woman on a mission. Where have I heard that before?* A memory washed over me. Of course. I used those very same words to describe Sharon on the night I met her.

***

Gettysburg College, 1995

We'd both attended a leadership conference at Gettysburg College geared to teachers in Pennsylvania. As with all summer nights, the sweltering heat affected everyone. As one of the organizers of the conference, I had my rounds to run. But for a little while, I stopped at the social dance prepared for conference attendees that evening. Newly-divorced, I found myself looking at the dance in a new light.

A movement caught my eye. A cute little brunette in a sleeveless blouse and blue jeans, which nicely showed off her narrow waist, moved toward me like a woman on a mission. Being a red-blooded American man, I could not help but notice how nicely she filled out her top. She half-walked, half-danced to the beat of the music. Very hard not to with the amps cranked up that high.

Do I know that woman? I rubbed my jaw and tried to recall who she might be and where she might be from. I'm very good with names and faces, but for the life of me, I couldn't remember how or even if I knew her.

She moved so fast I thought at first she might be trying to escape the building. I turned sideways to get out of her way. But instead of moving past me, she stopped right in front of me in the middle of the crowded doorway. Then, she tilted her head to look up at me—she only came to about my shoulder—and spoke directly into my face.

"Are you Joe? I'm sure you know my friend Patty. She's on the same committee you are. You know, in charge of things. Where is she?"

As I bent down to hear her over the noise, I could feel her breath on me—I rather liked it and lost my composure for a moment. I took a sip of soda to mask my surprise at the turn of events and pointed to the writing on my shirt.

"You mean the LDC, the Leadership Development Committee?"

"Whatever it's called." Her green eyes sparkled behind her glasses. I was drawn to her lips. Could have been the lipstick but I rather suspected it was the hot breath I felt on my face a minute earlier.

"Have we met?" I mouthed the words.

She held out a hand and shouted over the band, "Sharon from Erie."

"Joe from Pittsburgh."

She had a wide, open smile aimed straight at me. I felt like the only person in that room.

We attempted a bit of conversation but talking over the band took too much effort. I glanced down at my watch. Sharon's eyes followed mine. "Nice watch."

"Thanks. The color matches my eyes." I batted them in a very feminine way, which made Sharon giggle. I guess it would make a body laugh coming from someone my size and stature. *Don't look now but I just flirted.* I stole another look at my watch. As much as I was enjoying this talk, I had to end it. "I have to go now, but save a dance for me when I get off duty. Your friend, Patty, will be in soon."

"Okay," Sharon shouted back. Even then someone was leading her back onto the dance floor.

"Yeah, right. That will happen," I said aloud. *Not with Mister Old and Boring.* I walked out the door, suddenly relieved to have more duties to tend to.

I finished late. When I returned to the dance, the band was still playing, but all the women had taken to the dance floor. I stood for a while in the doorway, not wanting to seem overanxious for female companionship. A good friend of mine had cautioned me after my divorce. 'Be careful. Women can sense a man's desperation, and that's a big turn-off.' I stood there and wondered how not to appear desperate.

As I waited and tried to look nonchalant, shifting my feet, I found myself tapping my toes to the beat of the music. *Hope the next song is a slow one.* I looked over the bobbing heads on the dance floor. *There's that woman—the social butterfly from Erie. Hey, she sees me.*

She was waving to get my attention. I smiled, suddenly feeling a whole lot better. She held up her index finger to signal me to wait. Before the song finished, she arrived at my side. "Thanks for waiting." Sounding breathless, she tucked a stray hair behind her ear and patted the rest in place.

"You must be dancing with every Tom, Dick and Harry."

"How did you know?" She flipped her curly, sand-colored mop over her shoulder in a light-hearted gesture.

I started to enjoy myself. "I know everything. I'm

LDC."

"I did dance with Tom, Dick and Harry, in that order. That guy on the floor just now was Harry."

I inched closer. "You will now be able to say you've danced with every Tom, Dick, Harry and *Joe*."

Holding out my hand, I beckoned her onto the floor for my promised dance. The warmth of her hand seeped into mine as she grasped my fingertips. She skipped, kid-like, at my side as we tried to find some space on the dance floor. We found ourselves moving to the music. In a minute, she spun around and softly slid into my arms. That's when the band started to play one of my favorite dance songs, *Lady in Red.*

Strange thoughts came to mind—like how she danced the way a swan moved, gliding and effortless, so light-footed, she seemed to float on the smoky dance floor. *Joe, get a grip.*

"You and your husband must dance a lot," I whispered.

"I don't have a husband." She laughed and looked in my eyes as we executed another perfect turn.

My heart beat a little faster. I mulled that over for a few minutes, thoroughly enjoying myself. "Then you must dance a lot with your boyfriend."

"I don't have a boyfriend either."

Nice. Whoa. Joe. You've been divorced less than six months.

All the tables had been pushed back to one wall so the dancers could have more room. The crowd hung on the edges as they downed snacks and grabbed half-filled cups of beer and other beverages between sets. Some drinks had tipped out onto the floor. As I steered Sharon around a spill, I made a mental note to get a mop and clean up the messes.

We exited the dance floor after that number. Sharon

snapped her fingers and swayed to the music of the song that followed. A hint of her perfume lingered in the air between us. I wanted to ask what she was wearing but wondered if that would seem forward. Flirting. It had been more years than I could count since I remembered flirting. The moment passed and the song finished.

I let go of Sharon's hand and pulled an LDC member aside, "There's some spills that need cleaned up. Would you mind taking care of them? I'll get them the next time."

Sharon seemed itching to get back out on the floor. I cleared my throat. "Dance?"

Taking the dip of her head to mean "yes," I took her arm and led her to an empty spot. This woman twirled like she knew what she was doing. She moved easily in my arms, not once scuffing my shoes, trouncing my toes or kicking me. She never even stumbled during any of my double moves.

We dipped down almost to the floor and did another quick turn. I leaned in. "So, do you have any kids?"

"Two sons—Matt and Stuart." Her breath tickled my ear.

I smiled down at her. When she wrinkled her nose, I felt a ridiculous urge to touch it. Instead, I asked her what perfume she was wearing.

"Shalimar. One of my favorites." I felt a small thrill pass between us. Talking and listening to her came so easily, just like our dancing seemed effortless.

After the last dance, we took a moment to catch our breath.

"May I escort you to your room?"

"I'd like that."

We stepped into the early morning fog, comfortable but not touching now that we were no longer dance partners.

I slowed my stride to match hers. "How did you hear about the workshop?"

"My local president got me to come. She knew I wasn't at all interested in leadership but thought—uh, I could use a change." She left it at that.

"Not interested in leadership at a leadership workshop."

"I confess." She threw up her arms in surrender.

I wanted to kiss her at that moment but didn't do anything about it. I stayed on safe footing. "That is sacrilege."

We walked in silence until we reached her assigned dorm. "Thank you for walking me home," Sharon said, all nice and polite-like.

"Well…ah…er…I guess…maybe I'll see you around." *Lame. Very lame.*

I left her room and headed back to my dorm. It didn't

take much imagination as the fog swirled around me to think of myself wrapped in a cloud of her Shalimar perfume, and wondered if I'd ever see her again.

Oh, honey. I was lame then and I'm still lame. I'm so far from what you deserve. I can't even get a lousy meal for you or keep you from having to get this long operation.

Where is she? It had been more than four hours and I hadn't received a single update. Not one.

In a panic, I jumped out of Sharon's bed and reached the Nurse's station moments later. I barked, "What's going on with my wife, Sharon? Where the hell is she? Where have you taken her?"

"Sir?"

"Do you even know where she is? Sharon Belan!"

The nurse looked at me as if I were a lunatic. "You see, you've misplaced her! Can't even keep track of your patients!"

The nurse, frazzled by my accusations, searched frantically through the clipboards and then the computer. Finally, she said, "Mr. Belan, calm down. Your wife is still in surgery."

I looked at her suspiciously. "Are you just saying that? It's been far too long…"

"Surgeries take time. The doctors here are extremely professional and will notify you when she is out. I suggest you have a seat in the waiting room—"

"No thank you," I said stiffly, "I'll wait for my wife in her room."

I dragged myself back to the room and lay down. Every once in a while, I'd march over to the nurse's station again and pester them. I accused them of "misplacing" Sharon a number of times. Finally, I fell into a fitful slumber, awakening when the orderlies returned Sharon to the room in a drug-induced twilight sleep.

For a moment, I held her cold hand in mine and looked at her beautiful face, now marred by the cannula and breathing tube. She had IVs in both arms and a tube still draining her lungs. One of her lungs had collapsed from all the fluid in her pleural cavity. Silent tears trailed down my cheeks as I held her hand and prayed for God to remove her pain. "Just give it to me, God." I whispered.

Once again they kicked me out of the room to allow enough space to transfer her back to the bed. The eight hours we'd been apart felt like a lifetime. In the hallway, I stretched, smoothed out my wrinkled clothing and ran a hand over the stubble on my face.

God, if you're up there in heaven—and I know You are —bring us positive results from the surgery. We have a whole life yet to live. My shoulders slumped as I stood in the hallway waiting to see my wife again.

Chapter 3
THE RESULTS OF THE SURGERY

We heard a knock on the door in the morning. Sharon was still somewhat groggy from the operation, and I was in the middle of my third cup of coffee, pen in hand doing a Sudoku puzzle from the newspaper, when Dr. Clemente came bouncing into the room, once again followed by his interns. "A mighty good morning to you, Mr. and Mrs. Belan!"

"Uh, hello." I did some fast eye calisthenics to appear alert after the restless night I had.

"Are you and your wife ready for some good news?"

"Good news?" I took my wife's hand and said, "We sure are."

"We got it all!"

Sharon and I exchanged glances as the doctor went on to describe what he had done after he removed the diseased ovaries. "I took out all of the organs in the lower abdomen and washed them in a solution intended to remove any lingering cancer cells. Then I put everything back in its proper place and closed you up. Lastly, I inserted a small tube to help drain excess fluids."

"Damn. The way you explain it, Sharon sounds like a human-sized puzzle."

The doctor laughed. "Not quite that simple but that's the general idea." He went on in a more guarded voice, "All the cancer slides have come back from the pathology department."

We nodded, not really sure what that meant.

Doctor Clemente gave a wide smile and repeated, "We got it all." Jubilant, he turned to us, expectantly.

Sharon and I both sat in stunned silence. We couldn't

believe it.

Just like that our prayers were answered. All of the prayers of our friends, relatives and church had been answered.

"Hallelujah, God is good." I breathed.

Sharon hadn't moved a muscle. I put my arms around her shoulders and gave them a gentle squeeze, "Did you hear that, sweetheart? They got it *all*!"

"We'll need about three rounds of chemotherapy, just to be sure. We'd rather err on the side of caution. But all the tests came back negative."

I turned to him. "You are an *amazing* surgeon!" I pumped his arm up and down in the biggest handshake I could muster after a night of not sleeping.

Sharon still looked dazed but a smile lit up her face and she laughed out loud. "I'm not in an anesthesia-induced dream, am I?"

"Not you're not. You have my word on that," the doctor responded. He raised two thumbs up to Sharon and patted my shoulder, then bounced out of the room, ready to make more miracles come true.

The door closed with a sharp click. Alone, we hugged and kissed, and started making the rounds of calls to family, friends and church warriors.

***

That afternoon, we had visitors. I sat near Sharon's bed and watched her tell what had now become a humorous pre-operation "travel" tale starting from when the orderlies wheeled her out of the room for surgery.

"…and they dropped me off in the middle of some kind of abandoned corridor—I was pretty out-of-it but it seemed to go on and on without a single other soul…"

"Yeah?'

"Where did they take you?"

Having the rapt attention of her listeners, she continued, engagingly, "Yes, exactly! I'm like 'uh...where am I?' I lay there for quite awhile—I'm guessing a few hours—until a nurse came by. She asked, 'Ma'am, who are you?' By that time, I was even more out of it.

"'Huh?' I tried to look helpful. 'I—I'm a patient.' Wasn't it obvious? I was lying on a hospital cot.

'What's your *name*, ma'am?'

"'Ummm, if you don't know, I can't tell you. I feel kinda loopy, but I think I'm supposed to have an operation, um, now. I mean, awhile back.'"

I watched her hold court as her captivated audience chuckled and shook their heads in wonder. *She knows how to tell a good story. No wonder she's such a great teacher!*

"...Meanwhile, my doctor is standing in the operating

room, his gloved hands up in the air, saying, 'Where is my patient?'"

"No way!"

"The orderlies took me to the *wrong* hospital—in an adjoining hallway to another hospital—and no one could find me at first. Isn't that a hoot? They temporarily 'misplaced' me, can you imagine?"

My jaw tightened. Even though I had heard this earlier, it infuriated me that these orderlies—more like imbecilic Stooges—had just abandoned my wife in such a vulnerable state. My God! She wore only a paper robe and a light cover and wasn't even cognizant. I swore softly. *Take it easy, Joe*

"I accused the nurses of that very thing afterward—" I told my own forlorn tale of being neglected and out of the information loop. "But the doctor 'got it all' so we don't care about anything else."

Our family and friend clapped and cheered, "Yeah, he got it *all*." Our relief made us giggly.

Sharon had to stay at Magee for another week to ensure she was strong enough to eat on her own, and of all things, they wanted to be sure that she could 'pass gas.'

I volunteered to witness this feat, which earned me a rap on the arm from Sharon. A lady and quite private, all the attention on this natural bodily function embarrassed her.

Not me. I brought small candles to burn for the occasion. I unpacked the first one and set it on Sharon's breakfast tray. I'd just lit it when Nurse Ratched came striding in. Without slowing down, she snuffed the candle out with her fingers and thrust it back at me. "There will be no lighting of candles in this room, sir. It's an oxygen hazard." Without waiting for a response, she marched out of the room, very much in control of the situation.

I chased her down the hall and threw questions at her back, just as I had earlier. "How about a vanilla one? It's kind of like food. No? That's right. You're against food! What about a small scentless candle? Nothing? What do...?"

"No candles means no candles," she called over her shoulder, one hand on her hip.

I returned to the room and made a show of standing at the door, peering first to the right and then to the left. I pretended to get an all-clear signal. *Okay.* I marched over to Sharon's bed tray and pantomimed picking up a candle and snuffing it out. With my hands on my on my hips, I shook my breasts and made a very crabby face. "No candles means no candles." I strutted around the room snuffing out invisible candles and showing Sharon my crabbiest faces.

She giggled and held her stomach. "Don't make me

laugh, honey. It *hurts!"*

I stopped and said with a straight face, "Sorry, Shar. No candles now to cover your farting. Do your best but have compassion on me, your poor husband." With that, I grumbled about the lack of fun and festivities allowed in a room.

Sharon rolled her eyes. "I think we can follow the 'No candles regulation.' *Try* to behave, Joe." Her green eyes twinkled.

On Friday, just before the weekend, Sharon finally passed gas. I heard it and also observed her face turn red. *Mission accomplished.* Time to go home.

As I prepared to move her into the required wheelchair, we heard a light tap on the door. The woman there wasn't wearing any kind of nurse's uniform but she looked familiar. She sat down by the bed and talked to Sharon. "I'm so glad things went well with the surgery. I just need you to sign this form…" She handed her a pen but included us both in the kind smile.

My wife signed the paper. "Now I remember who you are. The lady who came to me right before my surgery."

"Yes, Lisa Stall. I don't expect you to remember my name, though."

"We're thrilled with the outcome of the operation by the head of your team, the great Dr. Clemente. Now we can get back home and pick up our lives where we left off," I said.

"Where's home?"

"Erie, home of the Seawolves, and beautiful Presque Isle."

"You're from Erie? I'm your neighbor. My whole family is from Edinboro. I even studied at the university there. Do you know it?"

Edinboro! Know it? How can I forget it! That's where

Sharon and I met up for the second time.

Edinboro, 1995

After the workshop in Gettysburg, I nearly put thoughts of the dance floor out of my mind—but not quite. It only took the wafting of perfume—didn't matter what kind—to bring back that Shalimar-filled night, two sparkling eyes and a small waist slender enough for me to circle my arms around.

After six long, awkward months, my ex-wife had finally moved out and on to her life in Albuquerque, New Mexico. Though I welcomed my newfound independence, the silence weighed on me.

Truth was, I was happy as hell to be getting away for the weekend.

On the road to the golf outing organized by members of the LDC in Gettysburg, I got a call and fished my cell phone out of my pocket. A gravely voice greeted me on the other end. "Where are you, Joe? I just rang your doorbell but guess what? No Joe?"

"Sorry, Burney. I'm on my way to Edinboro, in the northwestern part of the state. There's a golf tournament there."

"Just wanted to be sure you were okay. How ya doin' with uh, the divorce an' all?"

I shrugged. "Hangin'in there. Just keeping busy. My son's angry as hell at both of us … I'm waiting it out."

"Okay, Joe, have fun. Hope it brings something good to you."

"Thanks, Buddy. Nice to know someone's got my back."

By mid-morning, we'd all had our fill of golf and followed our rumbling stomachs to the picnic area nearby. I saw several familiar faces in the long line that curled around the pavilion. We had a mini-workshop reunion with the Gettysburg crowd as we waited. Finally, with a full plate, I scanned the tables for an empty seat. *I might just have to stand up to eat.*

"Joe! If it's not Joe from Pittsburgh!"

To my surprise, my dance partner from Gettysburg stood up and waved. "Sit here." She patted the empty seat directly across from her. Her mouth curved upward into a smile.

I saw a sweater lying there. "Looks like that seat is saved."

"Going, going, going…" She reached over and removed the sweater. "GONE!"

"All for the cheap price of…" For the life of me, I couldn't think of a funny punch line.

"A dancer extraordinaire!" She reached over and squeezed my hand. "Joe…" The top of her creamy white hand looked small over my darker large, clunky fingers.

Though her nails were clipped short, I saw that she wore clear nail polish—and no wedding ring.

"Sharon from…Erie. Do you golf, too?"

"Not today, I was just helping to organize and uh, getting together with some people from the workshop." Sharon looked fresh-faced and relaxed. *Lucky for me you did.*

I stood up. "I'm getting myself an iced tea. Can I get you something?

"I've already got a Coke, but you can bring me another."

With the Coke and iced tea in hand, I settled in and began to eat. I searched for a common topic of conversation. "Sharon, what grade do you teach?"

"Second. Such sweet children. They still love their teacher at that age." Her green eyes filled with affection for the children she taught. "You?"

"High school science—anything from physical science and biology to physics."

"Aaahh, I see. Biology, I can take. But physics!" She shuddered.

"Not so difficult. By that time, the higher-level students get into it."

Sharon and I waved to a number of people as we talked. Afterward, I was strangely reluctant to part ways. "You like sports?" She nodded and we meandered across the picnic grounds. After a lively game of team horseshoes, I looked around for another sport we could play, relishing the idea of prolonging our time together.

"Have you ever played bocce?" At her nod, we gathered a bunch of people to play. Soon, we had enough to make four teams. "Let's make this fun. I'll play against you now."

"Are you ready to take me on?" Sharon challenged.

She had a verve that matched my competitive spirit. I liked that.

"You bet! Now remember the objective is to—" I started to instruct.

"I *know,* get as close to that jack ball as I can." Sharon winked at me. "Bocce is my game."

In our teams, we jockeyed for the best positions. The swift-moving bocce game sped all over. As Sharon took her turn, I noticed the sun glinted off her hair making if look soft and smooth as it curled around her collar. Just then, she knocked my ball away from the jack ball. "Sorry." She shrugged, ever-so-innocently.

I looked away, hoping she hadn't noticed my attention. "I'll bet you are!" I shook my finger at her, playfully.

My next ball came nowhere near the jack ball. *Have to concentrate ... on the game.* She looked over at me. "Sun in your eyes, Joe?"

A few minutes later, I watched as she tossed her yellow ball underhand in one smooth movement. It rolled right next to the jack ball. She jumped up, high-fiving it with team members, and I once again saw that slim waist in action. She wore blue shorts and a t-shirt that showed off her trim figure. With my mind elsewhere, was it any wonder that her team won that Bocce game?

"Not only do you dance well, but you're an incredible Bocce player to boot."

"Awww…just lucky throws." She lifted an eyebrow. "Let me tell you about the time I took my second graders out to play bocce…"

The stories flowed out of us. Funny sports incidents led to funny classroom stories. We never seemed to run out of topics as we walked the picnic grounds.

Somehow that afternoon captured a playful side to me that I hadn't felt in some time. "Stand still!"I shouted, and swooped an open hand down to her shoulder. I drew a fly into my fist. "Got it!" I pretended to eat it.

"Ewww. Gross!" Sharon drew away from me and rubbed her palms on the pockets of her blue shorts.

How could a fifty-five-year-old Physics teacher behave in such a juvenile way?

After an awkward pause, Sharon's stomach growled. It took us both by surprise.

"Don't tell me you're hungry for flies too?"

"Ugh!" Sharon made a face.

Again, not the wisest move.

She changed the subject. "I know I ate a lot earlier, but I am actually getting hungry again," she admitted.

"Me, too. Well, no wonder. It's almost five-thirty."

"Really? You'll have to start driving back to Pittsburgh pretty soon, huh?" Sharon sounded disappointed.

"No, I'm staying at Sue Ellen's, one of the golfers at

today's outing. She was on my committee in Gettysburg."

"Yeah, I think I know who she is. About my height and athletic? PE teacher, if I remember."

"You got it. She said something about having a barbecue. Tell you what, if you can get me there, you're welcome to join us. There'll be a crowd, as I understand it." I took a slip of paper out of my wallet.

Sharon's mouth formed a surprised O. "Sounds great! My stomach is rumbling again. Let me see that address."

Sharon studied it for a moment. "I know exactly where this is."

"Is anyone expecting you?" I didn't want to monopolize her day—though I crossed my fingers, hoping she had the time.

"Not likely. My sons are off doing their own thing, and … no." She smiled but it faded quickly, leaving me to wonder what she almost said.

I jingled my car keys. "What are we waiting for then? I'll follow you."

True to her word, Sharon led me to Sue Ellen's place in short order.

"Glad you made it, Joe. How was your golf game?" She wore a cooking mitt and held a spatula in one hand while nursing a drink in the other. Her face looked tanned from a day in the sun. "Hey guys, this is Joe and …."

"Sharon," I supplied. "She attended the workshop in Gettysburg."

"Nice to see ya again, Shar. I remember now." Sue Ellen gave her a hug.

"She's had a few…" Sharon mouthed, waving her hand back and forth in front of her face.

Sue Ellen was speaking again. "Joe, lemme show you where you'll be sleepin' tonight."

I followed her to a room off the living room and

dropped off my bag. Back at the grill, I found Sharon chatting with one of the other teachers in her district. She motioned for me to join them.

"Help yourself to the food. Drinks are on the patio. Make yourselves at home. If you need anything at all, just ask." After a few quick introductions, she left us to our own resources.

Sharon and I talked for hours. As our voices grew hoarse, I yawned. "I don't hear any noise outside. I wonder if everyone's gone home?"

"Most likely." Sharon stretched out her arms and legs, her hands intertwined, feet crossed and toes, extended.

"The way you stretched there, you look just like a cat."

When she laughed, it sounded like "Pshhh."

"Don't hiss at me, now." I backed away in mock fear.

"Oh you." She closed her eyes for a minute.

"Look, I'm awfully tired. Do you mind if I lie down?

We can continue this conversation in my room. You can sit or lie down on the bed, however you feel most comfortable. Go to sleep if you feel tired, whatever."

"Okay."

We didn't have any of the awkwardness there would have been, had this happened thirty years earlier. But at fifty-five and forty-eight, respectively, we just wanted to talk and be comfortable.

Sharon sat, propped up by a pillow and dangled a leg over the side of the bed. "Tell me more about your life, Joe."

"That's a pretty big topic. You're gonna have to narrow it down a little. Half the night is already gone."

"Well, okay, tell me about where you live. Your place."

"I'm recently divorced. So, as you might guess, I now live in a bachelor pad."

"Uh-huh. Knew that." She paused, her face coloring.

"My friend, Patty, filled me in on those details."

"You … were fishing."

"I'm in the midst of a bad marriage now," Sharon said softly. "It's not that I don't love him. Well, I don't anymore. It's complicated. I guess everyone says that, though. His … uh, *behavior* is driving me crazy."

Sharon suddenly seemed very fragile. I had the urge to touch her. To comfort her? But it went beyond that. How I wanted to kiss her, to hold her.

She made a face. "The truth is, my husband is likely with a lady friend right now."

I stared at her. "Oh. A *lady* friend."

"Yep. It never seems to get any easier to say it. We're in the process of getting a divorce."

"I'm sorry." I wish I had more to offer her. *Divorce is hell. I ought to know. I've been through two of them.*

"Thanks. Humph. That's really only a little of the

indignity of our marriage…"

I watched her lips as she was speaking, almost

mesmerized. *If I just lean over, I can kiss her…*But I let the

moment slip from my fingers. We continued talking for a

long time. *You must either like me—at least a little. If not,*

you would've gone home.

Eventually, our voices gave out and we fell asleep—

fully clothed—on our respective sides of the queen-sized

bed. About four hours later, I woke up in pain from napping

at odd angles, twisted up in my clothes. I found Sharon

looking in my direction.

What is she thinking?

I felt Sharon's hand on my arm. "Honey, what are you

thinking? You ready to leave the hospital?"

I shook myself out of my daze. "Of course." I helped

my wife into the wheelchair.

"Here's your purse," Lisa said, setting it on Sharon's

lap. "Well, take it easy now. Enjoy your drive back to Erie."

She stood up, pen and clipboard in hand and waved good-

bye. From our open door, we could hear her heels click

down the hallway.

"I like her," Sharon observed. "She's a real

gentlewoman."

"Me too. Ready to roll, princess? This chariot is

headed for the exit."

***

Somehow, seemingly overnight, the weather had

changed from summer to fall. I stepped out the back door

of the house and a blast of crisp, cool September air hit me.

A few orange and yellow leaves from the maple tree in our

side yard swirled in the air and plopped onto the ground.

The sun highlighted a golden path through the carpet of

leaves that had already fallen.

Sharon called after me, "Apples, I'd like the biggest,

reddest apples you can find! I feel like making a pie."

I stopped and traced a large figure-eight in the leaves with my sneaker. "Are you up to that?" She was due for her first chemotherapy treatment soon. I wanted to make sure she didn't wear herself out.

"Honey, you just worry about finding the best apples you can." She paused. "I *am* getting stronger."

"Well, I'll bring some back but we'll have to see about the pie. Shall I get some cider, too? Maybe some doughnut holes?" *If we get cider, maybe you'll forget about the pie altogether. That won't be as taxing on you.*

She leaned against the door jamb, wearing footie pajamas and looking about twenty-five years old. *You look so young and beautiful.* My heart crashed against my chest. I consciously turned away from her and looked toward the car. I thanked God for sparing us. *Time with Sharon seems so precious now.*

I turned around again. "Babe, you up for a drive?"

"Thanks Joe, but it'll take too long for me to get ready…"

"I'm in no rush. I got all day. We'll, ah, make a trip out to Fuhrman's."

When she still looked undecided, I put on my obstinate face, raising my eyebrows in a ferocious Joe-scowl. But I couldn't hold it. "Come on, honey. You know you want to…"

"Okay, I'll be right out."

When we stepped out of the car and saw the familiar mill, I nudged Sharon. "You remember the first time we ever came here?"

She cradled my arm in hers. "Yeah, I talked you into it. Remember I said, 'Perfect day for a drive. Might be our last good day. The leaves are almost off the trees now.'"

The memory of that day washed over me.

Erie, 1995

"Perfect day for a drive where?" I finger-combed my gray hair and yawned, looking over my coffee at her—no telling what she had up her sleeve.

She had her crack-the-whip voice. "Thought we'd drive over to the old Fuhrman cider mill. I need some apples, and I'd love to show it to you. It's a beautiful, historic Erie landmark, about a hundred years old. I was also thinking we'd buy some cider. Then go to some doughnut shops, get one at each place, skedaddle to the car and taste test 'em with the cider. You in?"

"You bet!"

The cider mill did not disappoint with its rustic barn amid the maple trees, even though most of the leaves had fallen. Sharon played guide as we trampled through the golden carpet of leaves. The autumn sun warmed us as we saw different areas of the mill. The pungent aroma of apples permeated the place, making our mouths water.

"Mmmm! Smells *so* good, doesn't it?" She pulled me toward the store where we bought a bushel of apples and our own cider. Nothing less than a gallon would do but I would have bought more if she'd asked me.

"Come on. Time's a 'wastin,'" I waved her list filled with the names and addresses of doughnut shops she'd written.

"No rush. We have all morning," she reminded me in her gentle way. "Look at those clouds." She pointed to a clump of puffy white above. "They look like bears rolling on the grass."

I peered into the air. Clouds that looked like rolling bears? Nope, couldn't see it. Now, if she were to ask me

what *kind* of cloud, I could identify it as a cumulonimbus,
but bears rolling on the ground...

Sharon took my hand in hers and squeezed it. "Isn't
this fun, dear?"

Dear? Now *that* was almost worth pretending I saw
bears rolling in the grass.

The sunshine slid permanently behind, ahem...the
rolling bears. Out of the blue, the leaves skipped forward
along the ground. The air turned chilly. I tapped the list.
"Hey, I don't want to rain on your parade but it actually
docs look like rain. Don't you think it's time to move?"

She looked up and saw the sky turn dark.

I took her hand, and we headed for the car. As I closed
the doors, the rain pelted the windshield. "Just in time," I
laughed, heading for the first doughnut shop on the list.
Again and again, we'd dash indoors, make our purchase
and race back to the car. Water dripping from my fingers,

I'd fill our plastic glass a quarter full of cider and we'd take a bite of a doughnut before washing it down with the tart mixture. We sampled until we couldn't face another doughnut or a single drop more of cider. Together, we declared H & K Donuts the winner and headed home.

I carried the apples to her garage. "What are you going to do with a whole bushel of apples?"

"Did I ever tell you I had my own cider mill? I take it into school and teach a unit on it every fall. The kids make their own apple cider and write about the process. Boy, do they love it. That's what these apples are for."

Sharon constantly devised ways to give her students hands-on learning experiences. "The kids oooh and ahhh when the apples get all squished up and then, of course, no one can wait to taste the cider afterward. I think it's my favorite unit."

As I watched this lady lean against the garage door and

scuff rotting, wet leaves at her feet, I admired her more than ever.

Shar smiled as she held onto my arm. "I'm glad you talked me into coming today. It's early in the season and not too crowded. Can you smell those apples? Ahhh."

The leaves were just starting to fall today and we had blue skies overhead. No threat of rain or bears rolling in the grass as we walked around the old cider mill. Sharon was leaning heavily on me, so I slowed down. "You okay, babe?"

"Sure. I just feel a little tired. At this time last year I was getting my students ready to make their own fresh cider. I wish I were teaching right now. I miss those little seven- and eight-year olds. You know I do."

"I know," I said giving her a gentle, but big bear hug to infuse more strength and health into her slim frame. *It's only been a week since the operation.* "That'll come sooner

than you can spit dried pumpkin seeds across a table!"

She playfully pushed me away from her, "You crazy

guy!" Her voice sounded more energetic. "Joe, let's buy

some apples. I've decided to bake that pie, after all."

Chapter 4
SETTLING INTO FALL

The white block letters on the double-paned glass door read REGIONAL CANCER CENTER, with the hours posted underneath. We stepped inside. *This is it.*

At the end of the corridor, Sharon came to the entrance of a large room and surveyed it while I held her hand. With the mid-morning sun glinting through the slats of the white window blind, it didn't seem quite as scary as I thought it would. But what I thought didn't mean squat. It was Sharon's opinion that counted.

She paused. "It looks like one of those old-fashioned beauty parlors where all the busy-bodies used to sit under the very hot hair dryers for a spell and flip through pages in *Vogue* or *Better Homes & Gardens*. You know ... where the ladies shamelessly gossip as beauticians sit on stools giving manicures and pedicures."

I picked up a hand and inspected it playfully. "Hey Shar, I'll polish your fingernails and your toes. Just say the word."

She rolled her eyes. "Oh, you will? My toes? That's what I'm afraid of! With your clunky hands, I'll have polish all over my hands and feet, with the occasional bit on my nails."

My jaw dropped down. "Hmph. I meant—"

"...that I was a gossip?"

I was no match for my wife in her teasing mode.

Though the room held several brown leather recliners in a row, I realized that we'd never find a hair-dryer in this room. *Maybe not even hair.*

As if to prove my point, I saw that a middle-aged woman occupied the first recliner already. A red cotton scarf knotted in the back covered her head. Hard to tell how much hair she had or if she had any at all.

This sobered me. Despite all our teasing and joking, both of us knew the seriousness of coming here. Thank God the doctor had gotten all of Sharon's cancer and that the three rounds of chemotherapy served as a mere precaution.

Sharon's voice cut through my thoughts. "Joe, I can *do* this. What's three weeks of my life to safeguard my body? The military gives up a whole lot more for our country."

I pulled her toward me and tapped her once on the lips with my pinky, *"I'll* be your country. Repeat after me, 'I pledge allegiance to God and my country, Joe Belan.'" I needed her to safeguard me—more than she would ever know.

I helped her into the recliner and took her jacket from her outstretched hand.

"Pledge my allegiance to you? Didn't I do that five

years ago when we got married?" She eyeballed a lady who approached with several vials of blood stored in a mobile tray. The woman tied a thick rubber strap to Sharon's upper arm and was tapping it to find the vein. "You'll feel a little prick, dear, and a minute later, I'll be through." She winced as the lady did what she had to. Then we waited. When her white cell blood count was deemed high enough for her to withstand the chemotherapy, the soft-spoken technician returned to hook Sharon up to an IV.

I had one goal: distract my wife. "Shar, do you remember the first place I ever took you sightseeing in Pittsburgh?" I turned her face away from the IV. "It was a Saturday night…"

"How can I remember? We went so many places. Remind me." She winced in pain.

"After a full day of sightseeing downtown, we ended up eating dinner at the Sheraton Hotel on the south side, remember?"

Afterward, we crossed Carson Street and rode the Allegheny Incline to Mount Washington. I watched the twinkle of the city lights sparkle in Sharon's eyes. Once we reached the top, we walked arm-in-arm along the sidewalk, stopping at each of the scenic overlooks to take in the magnificent panorama of the city below us.

"Look Sharon, do you recognize that street?" I pointed to a spot where we'd walked earlier.

"It looks so different from up here," she marveled.

"It matters what you're looking at and from where." Somehow those words sounded all wise. Seeing Pittsburgh from Sharon's viewpoint made me see the Burgh in a different light.

"It all looked more beautiful." I finished up.

"Awww, you're a sweetheart." Her face grew reflective. "Remember when we went to the Benedum?"

"You mean the time we saw *Les Miserables*? Unfair! Let's not revisit that."

"Ha! You bought front-row seats two months in advance. You looked very handsome in your black suit and tie. I wore that emerald green cocktail dress…"

I headed her off. "In my defense, the auditorium was in almost black-out condition, lit up only when those fake explosions went off…"

"You fell asleep, and you were snoring!"

"Three things conspired to cause my downfall. My seat sloped down five degrees. The heat made me drowsy. The darkness put me right out."

"I tried to nudge you awake. But I couldn't control the cannon explosions. If only you hadn't jumped out of your seat when you heard them. Those poor actors forgot their lines! You're too funny." She poked me with the tip of her foot.

"Well, the book kept my interest. The play bored me to death," I muttered.

"Not to death, but certainly to sleep."

Watching the laughter spill out of Sharon made every inch of my red face worth the embarrassment that day.

Each day challenged us. Sometimes her low white cell blood count prevented her from getting treatment. When that happened, she needed a transfusion. Or, if she couldn't support the chemo, she'd receive blood serum instead. The chemotherapy also compromised her immune system. We couldn't expose her to crowds or even small groups of people. Bloating, one of the more embarrassing side effects she experienced, made her self-conscious and she refused to leave the house. Her face looked like that of a 200-pound football player.

One afternoon, she had another adverse reaction that upset her during the treatment. When I looked up from the mystery book I was reading, she seemed particularly frustrated and on the verge of tears. "Honey, my feet…"

"What's wrong with your feet?"

"It's like pins and needles."

Here we go again, another emergency! I scrambled out of the room to find the doctor. When I couldn't find him, I dragged one of the nurses with me. She asked Sharon some pointed questions and examined her feet. "Yes, as I suspected. This tingling sensation like your foot is asleep is one form of 'neuropathy.' Another form of it is simply pain. What happens, unfortunately, is the chemo damages or deadens nerve endings in the periphery—your hands or feet. I'm sure your doctor discussed this with you in preparation for your treatment. It occurs with nearly everyone who undergoes chemotherapy. Information overload, I suspect."

"Oh! How long do you think this will last?" Sharon

looked frightened.

"It's hard to say. It varies from patient to patient."

Sharon wiggled her feet and tried to bend her toes.
"What if it doesn't go away?"

The nurse patted her shoulder. "We have some therapy
that can help later."

"This feels very weird. But it's okay...it's okay."

I got ready to give my curled lip and mean Joe stare to
anyone who thwarted my wife. It killed me to see her suffer
like this. A vein pulsed on the right side of my forehead as I
fought to remain calm. "It's *not* okay."

Sharon's lips formed a thin, angry line at my outburst.
"Joe, getting angry isn't helping anyone, least of all me. I
need you right now."

"I'm sorry." I collapsed onto the chair beside the
recliner and buried my head in my hands. *How could I be
so selfish? I needed to safeguard my wife, not the other way*

around. "I can take the sickness. I can take the headaches. I can sit with you all day long. Give me any teacher's problem at Gettysburg. I can fix it. But I can't fix *this*. You've gone through so much already…"

She smoothed out my hair with gentle fingers. "Lay it down, Joe. Give it to God."

When we experienced these minor flare-ups, I'd remind myself we'd see better days. And they did come. By the time my birthday rolled around at the end of October, she'd finished her treatment. Right after that, Sharon went back to school full-time. In fact, she had been teaching throughout her chemo treatment with a substitute handling the hours when she received her treatment.

The day before my birthday, she came to the table wearing an olive green dress that brought out the green in her eyes and a shoulder-length, curly-haired chestnut wig.

"That shade of brown looks great on you." I cleared

my throat to draw her attention. "*I* picked that one out, didn't I?"

She patted the curls self-consciously. "Probably. It looks all right, then? Joe, remember tomorrow morning, we're going to Taki's to celebrate."

"I'm not going to forget my own birthday."

She slid the shoulder strap of her purse off the chair, threw on an olive jacket that went with the outfit and headed toward the door.

I put on my mean Joe glare. "What? I don't get a proper kiss this morning?"

"Too late. Gotta run." My glare didn't faze her. She blew me a kiss and hurried out.

I smiled. *Losing your touch there, Joe.* Actually, normal life felt pretty damn good.

October twenty-eighth dawned cold and rainy. But we got up early and headed to the restaurant to celebrate anyway, as we had every other noteworthy occasion for the past seven years. Just inside the door, Javina, the waitress at *Taki's,* waddled over to us. "What're ya celebratin' now, huh?"

Sharon pointed to me and said in a sing-songy voice, "It's his birth-day!"

"Happy Birthday. You the MAN! What a great way to start th' day! Y'all are in loooove! Make my heart go pitter-patter."

Javina had quickly become our favorite, but we knew all the waitresses, the manager and the owner. We felt like family as soon as we stepped through the door.

"C'mon now. Sit down right here." She pulled out a chair for Sharon and sat her down. "I'll get two coffees with cream and sugar—I know right well how ya likes it. Y'all are the only ones I know who looove celebratin' so much that ya come first thin' in the morning'"

"That's because we loooove to see you, our favorite waitress." I grinned. My birthday was off to a great start.

"Joe, I'm so glad we made coming here a tradition. You set up a good thing with breakfast."

"It's not me that made the choice. We both did. We ate here…dadadadah…the morning after…dadadadah…our first night together. It became *the* special place."

"Oh, you! Don't give me that drum roll. We didn't even do anything that night. We just talked. But later … in the great room, now that's where you need the drum roll."

***

Erie, 1995

Following my golf outing, and the barbecue at Sue Ellen's place, Sharon and I talked the night away. We fell asleep together—opposite sides of the queen-sized bed—

without even a kiss to mark the event.

I smiled over at Sharon. "Good morning, Sunshine." She looked beautiful with the early rays of sunlight shining off her hair.

"Good morning." Her voice sounded brisk, as if she were addressing her second graders.

"I gotta brush my teeth and find someplace to eat." I winced at how mundane my words sounded in comparison to the intimacy I felt watching her just moments ago.

"Bathroom is that way. I already did mine." She looked neat and tidy as she sat down to pull on socks and tie up her sneaker. The only evidence that she'd spent the night in her clothes was a wrinkle in her T-shirt I saw her smooth out. "Would you like me to show you a place for breakfast?" she asked, lacing up her other shoe.

"Sure. You know this area better than I do." I smiled over at her, hoping my breath wasn't too bad.

After writing Sue Ellen a thank-you note, we tiptoed outside. I opened Sharon's car door for her and waited while she snapped her seat belt. "For someone who has no interest in being a leader, you sure do an excellent job in leading me around Erie."

Sharon laughed—a delightful, unselfconscious, *pure* sound.

I winked, closing her door. "I'll be right behind you."

She stopped in front of a place called *Taki's,* a small restaurant with a robin-blue façade. "Best breakfast food around. They even say that on their sign." She pointed. "See?"

"Huh. Hope they live up to it. I'm starved." I swung open the door. "Ladies first."

A waitress ushered us to a table. Sharon hung her purse on the back of the chair and sat down. I double-checked to make sure I had my wallet and credit card, then took a seat.

Sharon picked up a menu. A mere thirty seconds later, she closed it.

"You know what you want already?" *I haven't even looked at the menu and she's ready to order!*

The waitress plunked down water glasses. Sharon took a sip and looked at me. "Take your time."

When the waitress returned to take our order, I let my date order first, as any gentleman would do: "I'll have two eggs over easy, two slices of crisp bacon, toast with grape jelly, hash browns, an orange juice and hot coffee."

My mouth fell open. *How could someone so slim put away that much food?* "I'll have the same, except do you have strawberry jam for the toast? And that'll be coffee with—" A glance at the table told me I had all the cream and sugar I needed. "That's it for me."

After the waitress left, I turned to Sharon. "Not hungry, are you?"

She laughed. The sound of her laughter made my heart sing. *How could I feel this way? I don't even know this woman, though I did sleep with her...fully clothed.*

The food arrived promptly and tasted great.

I signaled for the bill and the waitress returned. I crumpled my napkin. "Okay, you got me," I said as I handed her some cash. "*Taki's* is *the* place for breakfast. When I come back to Erie," I looked at my date, hoping that I, indeed, had a reason to return. "I'll come back."

Again, I held the door open for Sharon.

"What a gentleman. I like that."

"You can thank my father. He'd be happy to hear I've learned how to be a gentleman."

She turned sideways and gave me a look. Her green eyes sparkled with mischief, but she said nothing.

I raised an eyebrow. "What?"

The look was gone, replaced by an innocent smile.

Had I imagined it?

"There's your car," I gestured, pleased I could recognize it already, and walked Sharon back. Of course, I opened the door for her.

"A gentleman to the end." She rolled down her window and shaded her eyes to see me as I stood in the bright sun.

I could feel a lump forming in my throat. "Well, um, it's been good—"

"Joe, it's still kind of early. Do you have to get *right* back?"

"What's that?"

"I'm thinking…If you have time, I can show you Presque Isle and after, where I live."

Sunday morning. What the heck? I don't have to be back to Monroeville till this evening. "Lead on, fair maiden."

Off we went in our little two-car caravan to the beaches of Lake Erie. Then, to her house in Summit Township—neither more than fifteen minutes away.

When we arrived, I parked in the driveway and met Sharon in the garage where she parked her car. I announced, "I'm pretty sure you can get anywhere you want around Erie in fifteen minutes."

"You think so?" She looked amused.

"Seems like it. I have to clock it though. It's nothing like Pittsburgh."

"Hmm." As we passed some lawn chairs leaning against the wall, she picked up a newspaper lying on top. "Sorry it's so messy."

"Not at all," I replied automatically. To my astonishment, I found thick sheets of stainless steel eight feet by four feet bolted to the wall. I walked up and touched one of the sheets. Smooth. That material would never get a single dent. Stainless steel—strongest substance in the world. I whistled. *That's got to cost a pretty penny!* Question was, what was it doing lining the walls of a garage?

"That's my husband's, umm, 'handiwork' covering the drywall. He decided he'd like to set up a garage specially prepared, just for washing cars. Course, he needed something that water wouldn't damage. So, he found the perfect material at his place of employment—free of charge —if you get my drift."

"They *gave* all this to him?"

She shook her head. "I never asked. I thought it was better not to know. But they do sell this material in their product line."

I raised an eyebrow. *Was she saying he helped himself to it? Maybe he got a good deal on it.* "Worth a helluva lotta money. Got some nickel alloy in it." I looked at the large, heavy strips. It didn't seem like something a company would sell on the sly. "How did he get it out without anyone seeing?"

"I have no idea. I couldn't believe it myself."

Nodding, I decided it would be prudent to drop the matter.

A couple of garden tools leaned against the front wall. Aside from the tools, the garden chairs, and a hose wound on a spool, nothing but Sharon's car filled the garage.

She unlocked the door and led the way up some back stairs. "This is the house, be it ever so humble." As she neared the top of the wooden steps, she bent over and picked up a couple of *Family Circle* magazines. "Ugh. Sorry again. I didn't plan on having anyone see this place today."

"Sharon, you have a great place."

We passed through a white-framed doorway that led to

the living room. She scooped up a detective book and closed a women's devotional Bible before stacking them in a neat pile on an end table. "Tsk. So cluttered! Have a seat." She pointed to one of two tan leather sofas surrounding us.

The few knick-knacks she owned sat perfectly placed. I glanced around the room and saw that not one picture frame hung crooked nor did any lampshade tilt a single degree off balance. I wondered what she thought could possibly be out of place or messy. "Sharon, you should see my place. This isn't cluttered at all. All I can see is that you like to read a *lot*."

Sharon smiled. It reached her eyes, making them sparkle and then settled back on her lips. She changed the subject. "My house is a split-level ranch house. We have— *it* has—three bedrooms and a fireplace." Sharon swept an arm to indicate the fireplace in the den.

She picked up a picture frame. "This is Stuart, my oldest. He's twenty-five." She ran a hand over the glass of a smiling-faced man with light brown hair. She gently set it down and showed off another. "This one's of Matt. He's twenty-two and a junior at Edinboro University. Right now he's moving back in the dorm, getting ready for the fall semester. He's a good guy and a straight-A student, to boot." Sharon beamed. She took the liberty of showing me their rooms along with the rest of the house.

She reached out to a wobbly banister. "Careful," I cautioned.

"I *know*. This house needs some repair." She frowned as she stamped up the remaining two steps. "Hang on a minute." Sharon attempted, unsuccessfully, to tighten the screw with her fingernail.

"Hmmm. Sharon, just an observation but do you realize you've referred to your place as "this house" five times since we arrived?"

"What are you talking about?"

"I dunno. Just seemed kind of strange—not sure why —that you refer to your place as 'this house' kind of like you're angry at it."

"Oh. Well, it's not really a place I like much right now. My marriage is crumbling down around my ankles, so to speak," She lowered her voice. "In fact, my soon-to-be ex-husband is *fooling around* right in *this very neighborhood.* Yet, he doesn't want to give *me* the hell up. That man cannot make up his mind *who* he wants." Sharon stood very still, though her chest heaved in and out.

"What an SO—" I caught myself in the nick of time and dropped the B. I didn't want to curse in front of a lady. "I mean, that's low."

I know that feeling, and how quickly a home can become simply a house.

"My wife of twenty years decided that she wanted to live the lifestyle of a much younger woman. She asked for a divorce. Floored, I asked her why. She told me, 'You are too old for me. I'm bored.'" *Even now the memory of those words hit me in the gut.* I immediately regretted this confidence. What if Sharon thought of me as boring now? *Very dumb move.*

A heavy silence hung in the air. The hurt we each felt lay exposed. I thought I detected a look of empathy on her face but as quickly as it came, it went. She turned brisk. "Do you want to see the great room?" Before I could answer, she turned and set out in the opposite direction.

"Why not?" I called after her retreating figure. "Sure." I took big steps to catch up.

Retracing our steps from the porch, we climbed to the great room—a place easily the size of four garages.

I took in the stacks of drywall and rolls of insulation

tossed about. "Oh. But it's not finished." I turned in a circle to get a better look. It ended with me coming face-to-face with Sharon. We stared at each other.

"You know, I wanted to kiss you last night but was afraid of being rejected." I ran a hand through my hair. "May I kiss you?"

She whispered as she leaned into me, "What took you so long?"

I didn't answer. I simply placed my hands on her waist and bent down to kiss her. I watched her close her eyes and felt her arms encircle my neck. As I closed my eyes, her lips and mine met for the first time.

A rush of adrenalin and testosterone coursed through my body. We finally broke the kiss but did not move apart. We stood there holding each other, our breathing uneven.

I finally found my voice. "Wow. You can kiss and dance too."

"And play bocce," Sharon added, with that hint of mischief in her eyes again.

"C'mere." Why I said that when she was already in my arms was a mystery to me. *Geez, her presence affected me so much I didn't even know what I was saying.* Her waist seemed small and very feminine in my hands. It had been a long time since I felt this attracted to a woman. I didn't want to let her go so I pulled her even closer. I pressed into her—and she pressed back. This time I kissed her again without even asking permission. I didn't need to ask. The look on her face told me all I needed to know.

I continued kissing her for the next fifteen minutes, or as long I figured it took to drive anywhere in Erie. We broke free from that embrace, once again panting for breath.

"Whoooo-*that's* a long kiss." I exhaled. *I'd better calm down here.* "There are parts of my body that are working way harder than they have worked for the past five years."

She giggled, pulling away from me a little bit.

"I'm telling you the truth." My pulse was racing. I could feel a fire deep in my gut. "I'm not going to carry you to bed and ravish you." But I was thinking about it. Maybe in some part of my prehistoric brain, I was hoping that she would take me by the hand and lead me to her bed. Unfortunately, she didn't do that.

Don't blow it, Joe. Don't push. You don't want this to be a weekend fling. Be careful with her. This could work into a real relationship. The heady scent of her Shalimar perfume turned my legs to mush but I didn't pursue the direction of those thoughts. We both sat down amid the drywall. We talked for a long time but we ended up kissing and holding each other as much as we talked.

"Sunshine, I think it's time," I groaned at last.

"Time?"

"Time. For me. To leave." I punctuated each phrase with a kiss.

"Yes, I guess so." Her breath was still a little uneven.

We walked hand-in-hand to my car, trying to draw out my departure as long as we could.

"How do I get to the interstate?"

"Let me show you. Follow me." Sharon sighed, a long, drawn-out sound that told me she didn't want me to leave.

"Still following your lead, fair maiden." I called, just before I got into my car. Sharon backed out of the garage and I followed all the way to the throughway. At the underpass, she pulled off the road and parked her car. A minute later, she opened up the passenger door to my Chevy and slipped inside to say good-bye. Again. We said goodbye for another hour. I could have been to Grove City by that time.

"I'll call you as soon as I get home. Wait. Do I have your phone number?" I panicked. "I don't have your number." I dug into my pockets. Opened the glove box. *I always have a pen! This is not like me at all.*

Sharon unzipped her bag. "I have one. Remember, I'm a teacher."

"So am I." We looked at each other and burst out laughing. I realized she could see how flustered I felt. But I couldn't relax until I had her number in my possession. I couldn't bear to lose her over such a silly detail. We exchanged numbers then.

Sharon touched my arm lightly. "Don't lose it. I don't have your address, you know."

"Do you want it?" I would have given her any amount of information at that moment if it had guaranteed future contact.

Her smile told me she was flirting, even as she said,

"Of course."

As I scribbled it down, she asked, "So what did you think of the house?"

"It's a lot like mine—minus the six garages."

That brought more honest laughter. After a last kiss, she went back to her car but never actually got in. With the concrete road behind her and the underpass ahead, I thought she looked beautiful standing there. I could see from my rearview mirror that she was watching me as I drove up the ramp.

"Sharon and I have three special places already— Taki's, the Great Room and this I-79 underpass," I said aloud, drumming my fingers on the steering wheel. I felt absolutely alive.

Alive! Yes, and you said I was boring, Suzanne. Well, let me tell you, sweetheart, I'm plenty exciting when I'm motivated. I'm not old, or boring at all. You were at fault as much as me. Our marriage slowly turned into a marriage

of inconvenience, that's all.   I have enough adrenalin left

in my tank to get me safely home and then some!

I don't know how it is possible for every cell of a

man's body to be aroused. But all I thought about was

Sharon and me all the way home to Monroeville.

Just as I was turning into the driveway, a thought jolted

me: With the distance involved, what if this ended up being

a weekend fling? *Oh, God, I hope she hasn't changed her*

mind.

Javina plunked down the coffee and took our orders,

bringing me back to my very real birthday celebration.

Thank goodness you didn't change your mind! After the

waitress dashed away to deposit the ticket at the cook's

station, I leaned over and whispered, "I *love* this restaurant.

Happy birthday to me—no, to both of us! Shar, we made it

through your cancer scare. I am so grateful you're alive and by my side. *Never* forget that."

Sharon's face got all sentimental. "Joe, I feel the same way. This place is the *best!* It's all tied up in our fateful reunion that day seven years ago. And now, with everything we've gone through, this place means even more."

Javina served us quickly. As always, the food lived up to the faded letters on the sign. As I walked out of the restaurant hand-in-hand with my wife, I knew from experience that Javina would scoop up the big tip and tuck it into the top of her bra before she cleared the table.

***

With Sharon teaching her regular schedule with the second-graders, I took on the chores and the role of househusband again, which began with breakfast each morning.

"Sweetheart, breakfast is ready," I called into the bedroom.

"There in a jiff…"

Whether she'd come or not remained to be seen. Our new norm didn't vary much from the old. After we got married, I moved to Erie and we bought our own home. Always an early riser, I didn't mind preparing a hot breakfast for us each morning. In fact, as I had retired, it gave me something to do.

In our earlier days, Sharon rarely ate my breakfasts because she had it timed perfectly to get up and get ready for work. I'd tease her, "Have you got your make-up on yet?"

"Ha ha. You tell me." She'd stand beside the kitchen table and gulp down a glass of orange juice, daring me to guess.

I always said, "You look incredibly beautiful." She did.
I wondered why she spent so long putting on her face just
to look like she wasn't wearing any make-up at all. But
whatever she did, it worked.

She would tell me about her upcoming day as she
flitted about getting ready for school. Of course, she'd do
that from two rooms away. I struggled to catch what she
was saying as I banged pots and pans in the kitchen and
prepared breakfast. "You know I'm hard of hearing, honey.
What did you say?"

Again, I'd hear some indecipherable reply. "Shar, I
can't hear you unless you come into the kitchen."

Most mornings, she'd ultimately breeze through the
kitchen, grab a piece of buttered toast and her car keys,
give me a kiss, and quick-step her way to her car.
Sometimes we exchanged blown kisses as she backed out
of our driveway.

My days consisted of meal planning, shopping, doing crossword and Sudoku puzzles, and snacking continuously. I tidied up the house and even vacuumed. In her absence, I watched old VHS movies and newer ones on DVDs.

During a serious discussion one day, she sat me down at the kitchen table, took my face in her hands and in her most "I'm-concerned-about-you" voice said, "I'm worried about you sitting here home alone all day with nothing to do except play with your puzzles and watch TV. You're going to turn into a movie couch potato. I want you to get out of the house and go golfing."

One of the most difficult things that I ever had to do was to keep the smile off my face as I cast my eyes downward. I tried to create a sad, disappointed expression and mumbled, "Do I hafta?"

Needless to say, she successfully kicked me out of the house to go golfing. When I shared this story with my golfing buddies, they gave me "You-are-the-luckiest-man-in-the-world" looks. "I know. It's like dying and going to golf heaven!" I gloated.

As life returned to normal, one aspect changed—Sharon's hair. Of course, we expected the hair loss. But accepting it intellectually differed drastically from facing the reality. Sharon always took time with her hair. The expression, "A woman's hair is her crowning glory," fit her well. To lose it meant losing part of her identity. At first, she took it pretty well. But the more she lost, she more it hurt to see herself in the mirror.

"Aww Sharon, it's okay," I murmured, holding her close. "Don't worry. I'll buy you eight wigs. We can get red, brown, black and blonde-colored wigs."

"But I just want my own hair," she whimpered.

I continued as if she hadn't spoken. "We can choose four long-haired styles and four short-hair styles. That way you can see how you look and fit the style to your mood."

She stood, motionless, her hands clenched to her sides. "You don't understand."

"Well—" I thought fast. "Think how this will spice up our sex life. You can be whoever you want to be." I raised an eyebrow suggestively. "Or … maybe I can. One of those wigs could suit me just right … and Fabio will put in an appearance." I pursed my lips.

"Oh, you, get out of here." Sharon gave me a wan smile.

Ultimately, we purchased four very conservative wigs in similar shades of brown. We also bought a mesh cap that fit under her wigs because the stitching scratched her tender scalp.

Sharon took meticulous care of these hairpieces, shampooing them regularly. Real hair wigs required a special, expensive shampoo, and synthetic hair took a different, slightly less expensive kind. First, she would soak

the wig in a solution. Then she'd wash it in the appropriate

shampoo. After that, she'd pat it dry with a soft cotton

towel. Finally, she let it air-dry on one of the Styrofoam

heads we bought.

Although I supported my wife to the fullest degree, I

have to admit, life in the Belan household rendered me

speechless at times. Like when I entered the kitchen in

search of my favorite popcorn bowl. I found it all right. But

not in its place. There it sat on the counter with one of

Sharon's wigs soaking inside, looking every bit like a

drowned rat.

"Sharon!" I screeched and pointed as she ran into the

room. "That's blasphemous!"

"Oh sor—well, if I weren't bald, you would find your

favorite popcorn bowl empty, now wouldn't you?"

After several surprises like this, I began to pray

between fits of laughter that Sharon's hair would grow back quickly.

The wig saga went on. One day, Sharon came home from a Saturday outing with a teaching colleague. Her wool hat was askew and her cheeks were red from the cold. "Look at this rock, honey." She pulled off a glove and smoothed it with her hand. "Isn't it a beauty?"

I stared at her. "Another one?"

"Well, Linda and I were driving along deep in conversation about our problem kids when I told her to pull over to the side of the road. It all happened so quickly, she got frightened and asked if we had a flat tire. I told her of course we didn't. I just found the perfect rock to add to our collection." She thrust it at me with a triumphant smile.

"Shar. You know it's illegal to take any rocks from the side of the road." I tried to keep a serious face. She had never seen anything wrong with uprooting a special rock regardless of its size or location. "Out in the middle of nowhere? Who would want a rock like this except for me?" was her standard reply.

"It won't hurt for our rock collection to get a little bigger. This one is a special type of igneous rock. And it looks like the wig I wash in your popcorn bowl." She giggled.

I picked up the rock and looked at it from several different angles. "You know, it does. These look like the bangs and here are the waves down the side."

"I *knew* you'd see the resemblance. It's a sign! My hair's going to grow back for good. Where shall we put it?" She zipped up her parka and pulled her gloves back on then wandered slowly around the yard, seeking just the right spot to place her wig-rock. "How about next to the one we found on our trip to the Cleveland Rock and Roll Hall of Fame? That's right outside the kitchen."

"That'll work."

As long as it's nowhere near my popcorn bowl.

Chapter 5
ROOTING FOR THE STEELERS

November brought cold weather to Erie, Pa. The Pittsburgh Steelers had sailed through pre-season games and kicked it up a notch with quarterback Tommy Maddox at the start of the season. But after five consecutive losses, the Steelers began to flounder in the competition.

Diehard Steelers' fans, Sharon and I had season tickets to all the home games. For the past seven years, we took to the stands and rooted for our favorite team, win or lose. At the start of each season, we wore Steelers jerseys and shorts and added layers as it got colder. By season's end in late December, Sharon bundled up in a floor-length heavy coat, gold and black scarves and mittens along with a snowmobile outfit. I teased her every season about how she hated the cold but braved it for the Steelers.

Unfortunately, the Steelers team lost its star fan at some games during the 2003 season.

"I'm going to have to sit this one out, hon. I'm so sensitive to the cold right now. And my hair…" She made a pitiful face.

"I understand. Do you need me to stay home?"

"Are you kidding me? We paid a fortune for those tickets! I'll just hunker down on the sofa here with a blanket and watch it on TV. You get over to Heinz Field and we'll compare notes when you get back."

I knew she'd kick me out. Just like with my golf game. Of course Sharon and I always looked for ways to make each other happy. And the Steelers sure fit the bill! But as I glanced over at the empty seat next to me on my drive to the stadium, I missed her. On game days, we never had a break in conversation. I'd have to say, 'Sharon, hang on to that thought. I'm listening but I don't want to miss my turn off.' It had been that way from the start when we discovered our mutual passion for our Steelers.

Pittsburgh, 1995

Although we'd only had two "official" dates, they'd been intense and lasted a weekend each time. This time, Sharon had come to Pittsburgh to spend more time with me. We hit it off—majorly. As our time drew to a close, we sat together on the sofa…

Sharon leaned over and touched my leg. She was holding my hand, saying, "This whole weekend has been wonderful. It's early days but still…I feel…we connect."

"Really? I feel that way, too! Shar, I've been thinking this weekend—and I know this may seem sudden—but I just have to put it out there." She gave me a hard, questioning look.

"I have something *important* to ask you."

Suddenly, she crossed her arms. She coughed as if she

had a tickle in her throat she couldn't get rid of. I pulled something out of my back pocket and hid it behind me, then knelt down facing the sofa. Her eyes got very round and big. She blinked and did a double-take, craning her neck to see what I was hiding. I gently guided her attention back to me.

"Sharon, will you….go to the Steelers' games with me? I have season tickets so I guess what I'm asking is, do you want to go to *all* the games with me—the *home* games, that is?"

As I placed the book of tickets in her right palm and curled her fingers around it, she burst out laughing. "Joe, get outta here! You got me…are you serious about the tickets?"

I nodded. "Never been more serious in my life." I just hoped she wouldn't ask why I had the extra tickets. Things like that were better left unspoken—the past should stay in the past.

Her eyes traveled from the tickets in her hand back to me. Her mouth formed a big "O," as if she grasped the significance of what I was asking—moving to the next level in our relationship.

Although I'd been hatching this plan since the day before, I hadn't thought through the ramifications of her response. I was just riding the crest of excitement and didn't want this feeling to end. Even though my proposal came in the form of Pittsburgh Steelers' season tickets and this was a light-hearted gesture to make her laugh, I realized then just how much I wanted her to accept.

"Yes!"

The marvelous word ricocheted around the walls. Sharon said yes? She said yes! *Season tickets for you and me and the Pittsburgh Steelers.* All of a sudden, fall just got a little more interesting.

She danced in a circle, snapping her fingers and singing. "Who's gonna go to Steelers games? I'm gonna go the Steelers games." In a normal voice, she said, "Seriously, I *love* the Steelers."

I got off my knees. "Well, that was worth me making a fool out of myself. Now we know we're both diehard Steelers fans. What if I'd gotten rejected? Ah, my poor pride."

She rolled her eyes. "It was a rather, a-hem, unusual way of asking me out for a whole lot of dates. That took guts. At first, I was like…Oh my God, no! Please, don't let him be asking me to marry him on our second real date! I was scared there. You looked so serious."

I laughed. "Got your attention, you have to admit."

"You *did*. I like a good sense of humor. Just don't scare me like that again or I might faint on you."

I thrust my hand out. "Well, you scared me getting in

so late Friday night. So I guess we're even. Shake?"

She held out her hand. Instead, I leaned over, turned it and kissed the top.

"Oh, you're good. You tricked me." She shook her head as if to say, I can't trust you anymore, can I?

"I did." I sank into the sofa. She sat close by, her leg touching mine. I needed to focus here. "Okay, you know that the Steelers play next weekend? It's a one o'clock game. Why don't you come Saturday morning? You want to go shopping with me or should I do that on my own?"

"Just think of it as part of our date," Sharon joked. "Long-distance dating sure seems to speed things up, doesn't it?"

"It does when the two people in question are so close." I gave her a gentle look, a little afraid that I would appear too smitten.

She leaned over and cupped my face with her hands,

then drew me into a kiss. When the kiss ended, we both drew apart, somehow embarrassed but not sure why.

I coughed. "We can get the tailgating food that morning. After that, we'll get the equipment squared away." Already, I was mentally putting together one of many lists.

She peered over her glasses at me. "Hang on. This might be getting off the subject, but who do the Steelers play against for the season opener anyway?"

I thought for a minute. "They're playing the…"

"Detroit Lions!" Her green eyes sparkled as the name came to her.

"That's exactly right. I can't believe you knew that."

She shrugged her shoulders as if to say why-shouldn't-I-know, but the smile that tugged at the corners of her mouth betrayed how pleased she felt.

I'm sure I had a silly grin on my face. *Seemed to be*

doing a lot of smiling in the last couple of days.

"How about if I go to Erie on Friday, we fool around for a little while—" I wiggled my eyebrows suggestively "—and we drive back on Saturday morning to pick up all the food? After a good night's sleep, we can be ready to leave for the stadium by about five a.m."

"A good night's sleep? Ha!"

"Well, relatively-speaking…"

"Drive all the way to Erie, then turn right around and go back to Pittsburgh the next morning? Spend *aaallll* day shopping and getting ready for the big game then leave for the stadium at five a.m.? Are you nuts?" She reached out as if to choke me, "Aaaghh!"

"Going to a Steelers' game is a bit of a culture shock, huh?"

"It has nothing to do with that. Just figuring out the easiest plan. Okay. I'll drive myself to your house after work on Friday. Once I'm here—or maybe before—I'll prepare whatever side dish will go with the food we take. That's that."

Ah, a taste of her independent streak. I realized I'd have to quit being so high-handed with my ideas—no matter how well-intended—and start making plans ... together.

The following weekend, she arrived, psyched for our first Pittsburgh Steelers outing together. Casually dressed in a pair of worn blue jeans and a t-shirt with the slogan, "Mill Village Elementary, It takes a whole village to raise a child" emblazoned across the front, she got out of the car and tossed me a Nerf football. "Brought you a little something."

"Whew! Got it. Did you bring me anything else, like a hello kiss?" I threw the ball back.

"Think I can rustle one up." She said, faking a pass

with the football. The game was on and I finally tackled

her in the yard. We rolled on the grass and kissed. The sun

spilled across the grass, warming and blinding us at the

same time. "Kind of missed you this week," I said, tugging

at her hair.

"You did? It *was* busy—but I think I might have

missed you too."

We lay on the ground, talking and catching up with

each other until the air cooled and the sun filtered red

through the trees and finally set.

"Ugh! These mosquitoes." I pulled her up. "Tonight is

for us…if you know what I mean. Tomorrow and Sunday

are for the game. Deal?"

"Deal."

The next morning, the alarm went off at five. After

some eggs, toast and very hot coffee, I gave her the

lowdown of what getting ready for a game involved in my

book. "Just so you know, my preparations for attending any Steelers game are pretty much like the Allies preparing to invade Europe on D-Day." I rubbed my hands together. "Let's get started."

She whistled, as she took the notebook I handed her.

"I'll watch the morning weather as you read through the lists."

Ten minutes later, she looked up. "You sure you got everything?" She looked concerned.

"Well, I've been doing this for years—" I looked over her shoulder to see what I could have possibly missed.

"I see everything but the tickets down here." She tapped at one of the pages and grinned.

"A diehard fan like me would never head out to the stadium empty-handed," I assured her.

"Whew! That's a relief." Her eyes twinkled. "Season tickets don't come often to this diehard Steelers fan."

With the shopping and packing done, I suggested we start loading up the truck. I situated things the way I always do to maximize space. "I'll be right back. Just want to get something to wipe down the coolers." I switched on the light in the laundry room and went through the basket.

I returned with a cloth and reached up to swipe the condensation off the cooler. "Wait a minute, something is different here." I stared at Sharon. "Did you move some of the stuff around?"

"Me? Seems you've got it all well-arranged." Her voice sounded innocent. "Oh my. Look at the time. Can we call it a night? This nearly-fifty-year-old body is bushed."

I raised the tailgate and locked it in place. I knew she'd changed my set-up but she looked so damn cute with that innocent smile, I let her believe I thought I was mistaken. "I guess we're done here." Besides, something more pressing claimed my attention. "You're … bushed?" I raised a brow.

"I suspect a shower will rejuvenate me."

We awoke about four-thirty in the morning. We ate a skimpy breakfast to get us moving. Then I handed her my vintage Terry Bradshaw, number 12, jersey to wear. Although it was somewhat big, she put it over her blouse anyway. The last thing we did was brew a strong pot of coffee for the road. I shoved the thermos between us. "We need this up front today."

"Ah—coffee. I could go for a second cup." As Sharon climbed into the truck, she turned to survey the full-to-brimming load we'd packed. She hummed a few lines of the *Beverly Hillbillies* off-key, and started singing. As we pulled out of the driveway, any neighbor awake at that time of morning surely heard us belting out a new version of the song, paying homage to the Steelers. We laughed like teenagers, as if we didn't have a care in the world. *God, this is crazy and fun! This woman is so easy to just BE with.*

"I *like* singing with you, Joe." She ran her hands through her hair in an unselfconscious gesture and let them fall to her side before taking a deep breath. "I'm wide awake now."

We got into the stadium parking lot early. "Quick. Let's unload the truck. We need to save some spots for our friends. Spread it out. We've got eight carloads of people coming."

As the group arrived, I made the introductions. My pal, Burney, shook her hand warmly. "Welcome to the carnival, Sharon. You're gonna loooove these games and tailgating parties. We always have a blast." One of the guys blew a horn and shouted, "Go Steelers! All the way to the Superbowl!" Cheers rose and more horns sounded. From the onset, she fit right in. It helped that she knew a lot about the Steelers. But even if she hadn't known a thing, my friends would have welcomed her on board. Already, they were sharing insider jokes with her. *Even the laughter sounds sweeter with Sharon by my side.*

When the parking row filled up, we moved our equipment into the road between the rows of cars. I pulled out the Nerf football and tossed it to her, "Hey, catch."

She tossed it back, and I had to chase it. As I bent over to retrieve it, I said, "No fair, I am operating on just a few hours sleep here…"

"Excuses, excuses."

When we tired of that game, Sharon tucked the Nerf into a bag. "Who's hungry besides me?" she called out. I remembered how much she could pack away. Eager to please, I opened a cooler to prepare our first meal.

Later, we left the warm circle of friends behind. I took her hand, and we took off. "Let me show you around."

"What an operation. Look at all those flags. There are tents and even some home-made toilets with—are those showers?"

"No, they just use shower curtains for privacy."

"Huh. What's that long trailer used for?"

"That's a flat bed trailer. Do you see the DJ? He's setting up now. He'll play Steelers songs all day long."

Sharon elbowed me. "Joe, is that a hot tub? It *is*! There are a couple ladies in their bikinis sipping Margaritas in there. Go figure." Her attention moved on. "Oh, there's some kind of moving truck or something. What's that for?"

Reluctantly, I pulled my eyes from the buxom beauties in the hot tub to where she was pointing, earning me a light smack on the back. "Stop that." She gave me her stern teacher look.

"Yes, ma'am. Can you see that huge screen TV?"

She craned her neck to see. "There? Yep."

"They'll play re-runs of past Steelers games for awhile. When it starts, they'll show all the live action televised."

As she clutched my arm asking questions, I found myself sharing little known facts and personal stories of encounters with the players over the years. *It's gonna be a great season!*

As we walked around, we struck up some conversation with the Lions fans.

An enormous, big-bellied muscle man with tattoos plastered up his arms passed us. "Who *you* rootin' for?"

"Steelers, through and through can't you tell?" I dropped Sharon's hand and punched my fist in the air. "Go, Steelers!"

"Don't count on 'em winnin.'" The girl with the tattooed man swung her long, straight black hair in disdain. "Lions roar this season."

"That may be but this year belongs to the Steelers."

Sharon rushed to defend her champs.

"With Barry Sanders—greatest runnin' back of all time—you are mistaken."

Sharon countered, smiling sweetly. "Barry Sanders is truly amazing. In our defense, we've got Rod Woodard, all pro cornerback."

"*Looove* Detroit. And the team isn't half-bad," I interjected, affably.

Both women stared at me as if I had had spoken out-of-turn.

"I'm just keeping the peace on this beautiful sunny morning."

The tattooed man high-fived the girl with him and they walked away with a friendly wave. "Enjoy the game."

"You, too," I called. I turned to Sharon, "The Lions fans behave well, unlike fans from some of the other teams."

She rubbed her hands together. "Really? It's such a thrill to meet fans of both teams."

We wandered into the stadium about noon, an hour before game time. Sharon shielded her eyes from the sun and looked onto the playing field. I dropped an arm around her shoulders and pointed. "That's where the Steelers will come out."

Our seats were located in the last row of the stadium, right on the fifty-yard line. We looked up at the press box above our seats where NFL photographers, along with film crews for the Steelers and the Lions, snapped their press photos.

Sharon eyed the activity with interest. "I'm so glad we have these seats."

During the singing of the National Anthem, we took off our hats and stood, hand over heart, our voices joined those of fifty-five thousand other fans that filled the stadium. Sharon leaned over close so I could hear her as she whispered, "That sounded magnificent."

"I know. It makes my eyes leak every time," I whispered back.

After the action started, our eyes were riveted on the players; neither of us spoke much. The first quarter finished, and we were well into the second one when I realized how much more I enjoyed the game than in years past. *How wonderful it is to watch a game with someone who's really interested in what's happening on the field.* "You're amazing. You watch every play."

She didn't take her eyes off the field. "I told you I liked the Steelers, Joe. I watch them on TV all the time."

The center snapped the ball back to the quarterback. We stood up, screaming our lungs out. "Go, Slash, go!"

"Look! He's got blocking. Go! Go! Faster!"

On my feet as the adrenalin poured out, I shouted,

"Slash is the fastest quarterback. He's going to make it! Look at him Look!"

"Whoo-hoo! Touchdown!" she shouted.

It was a close game with the score ending up, 23-20, our favor. Sharon and I stayed in our seats, caught up in the Steelers' win, discussing various plays. Our conversation blew me away. A woman who I could actually have an intelligent conversation with about a football game. I glanced at the program in my hand. "Next game is with the Houston Oilers."

She picked up her sweatshirt and took a step down the bleachers. "The tickets are only for home games, right? I guess we'll have to see that one on TV." She made a face.

Almost everyone had cleared out of our section, so we had no difficulty getting down. By the time we got to the bottom of the escalators, most of the fans had dispersed to their tailgating sites. Everybody was celebrating.

The gang had gathered back at my Ford Explorer, waiting for me to unlock it and get the food and drinks out. "'Bout time!" someone shouted. "I'm ready to eat my shirt."

I unpacked some shrimp and held them up for Sharon to see. "Some shrimp to celebrate our first Steelers game together."

"Oh, that's so sweet." She caressed my arm.

"Well, I'd say it's time to throw 'em on the grill and celebrate."

Two or three hours later, we packed up our gear and headed home delayed, as usual, at the Squirrel Hill Tunnel, which was jam-packed with other Steelers fans trying to get where they needed to go. "It won't be long now. We should be home in about ten minutes." I looked over at Sharon. "So how was that for the start of the season?"

"Wow. Fabulous. Except poor Rod Woodson. Tearing

his ACL like that. He's gonna be out the whole season. If only Barry Sanders hadn't faked him out!"

"Yeah, tough break."

"But I can't wait for the next home game. It's completely different watching it *live*." She looked like she could do it all over again.

Just wait til the adrenalin wears off. I knew from experience how fast energy could drop.

With the Parkway clear, we arrived home a few minutes later. "Home sweet home."

I started my post-game ritual of putting all the perishables in the fridge, and the equipment back where it belonged. Sharon pitched in, and we finished in no time at all. Covered with grime, smells of smoke, sweat and food, we showered together, another novelty in a day of firsts for us.

Refreshed, we hopped into bed around ten o'clock.

"We just devoted seventeen hours to a three-hour football game," I marveled.

"Mm-hmm." Sharon's eyes were closed. Finding her on the verge of sleep, I held her in my arms. She would wake in the early morning for the two-hour drive back to Erie in time to greet her second-grade students for a new week of classes.

On Monday evening I called Sharon back in Erie to ask her how her day had gone. She grumbled about being rushed and sounded tired. I felt guilty. I hated the idea of her making the long drive home alone. "Is it too much?"

"I wouldn't change it for the world. I'm fine. Besides, I've made it this long on my own." She sounded slightly annoyed.

"Well, I just worry…"

I was no dummy. I backed off.

As I pulled into Steelers territory this morning without

Sharon, I somehow missed her more than ever. I hoped she would feel better and get to come to the other games, even if our team weren't playing too hot. I glimpsed Burney and a few of the guys in the crowd. They huddled near a large grill someone had set up. When I opened the car door, a fierce November wind hit me and whistled around the busy lot. I could see my breath fog up in the air. I zipped my Steeler parka up a little higher and pulled my knit hat down over my ears. *Damn glad to have my thermal gloves with me today.*

Burney clapped me on the shoulder. "Good to see ya, Joe. How you holding up? You've had your share of difficulties lately."

"Things are getting better, Burney. Soon, all this will be behind us."

"You guys sure are hangin' tough. Ha! Tougher than the team is doing this season, I might add. Bunch of wusses." He looked disgruntled. "Sharon's even made it to several of the games this season. I don't know how you do it."

Me either. It's Sharon's resilience. Her faith.

With a winning score of 28-15 over the Cards, fans left the stadium pumped. I didn't even wait for the crowd to go down as I normally would. I wanted to see something.

A couple years back, before Sharon and I got married, when the Steelers were finishing their new stadium, I got a letter in the mail informing me if I wanted to retain rights to our season tickets, I'd have to purchase a seating license. Of course, I followed through with it. It came with a perk— a brick with our names on it inside of Gate A. When the new Heinz Stadium opened, we were one of the first thousand fans to hover over our brick. We touched it reverently, excited that we had become a part of Steelers history.

I found it again. I cleared off some damp leaves that clung to the brick and read the words inscribed on it. "JOE AND SHARON BELAN." We knew we belonged together even before we officially got married. As Sharon would say, "*This* is a good sign."

I breathed in the crisp, cold air and fell to my knees. *Thank you, God, for bringing us together and packing so much into our relationship already! God, the same clay that physically contains our joint names, symbolically holds us together. It's Your clay, Your adhesive that binds us as ONE. Thank you for this physical sign of Your will in our lives.*

What? How did those thoughts get in my mind? I jumped up and hurried back to the car. I could hardly wait to tell Sharon what God had revealed to me.

Though the air around me felt about twenty-five degrees, the inside of me felt the sunshine of our love burning strong.

Chapter 6
FOOD, GLORIOUS FOOD

By the time Thanksgiving rolled around, we wondered if we'd have a good holiday or not. Sharon had her share of weak days yet. She still had bouts of residual vomiting from the chemo in her system. I saw her hair come out from time to time as she leaned over to throw up. She couldn't seem to get a consistent body temperature, so she alternated between burning up and having the chills. We never knew how she'd feel, so we couldn't plan ahead of time. Teaching took up most of her energy these days. What remained, she channeled toward feeling better. Our day-to-day reality kept us from doing anything extra though we held up the façade of energy when we had visitors. We didn't want to dampen anyone's holiday.

We asked each other how much effort we should

devote to the holiday and how much we should leave for self-preservation. One afternoon Sharon suffered a terrible attack of diarrhea. She turned to me. "Ooooh." She pressed her stomach with both hands and bit her lip. "Should we try to cook this year?"

"I don't know. Not if you are having that problem."

Shar loved spending time with her family, but we had a lot of variables to contend with, and Thanksgiving was just five days away.

Stretched out on the sofa later that night, I broached the topic again. "Babe, I think we should forget the holiday hassle this year. Simplify, that's the key."

Sharon planted herself next to me. "I'm reconsidering. Joe, you're really quite the chef, and you love to cook…"

"Oh no, appealing to my culinary skills is a waste of time—"

She jumped up and passionately pressed her fingers to

her lips and made a kissing sound as her hands opened up. "That spaghetti and veal parmesan dinner you put together the first time I ever visited you! Magneefico!"

"Ha! You Italianos! I didn't jus' prepare za dinner zat night, I prepared a whole veezit. Za top chef know how to plan for egzactly za right ambiance, and bring za totall package together."

Sharon laughed. "You call that a French accent? Ay, Marco Polo! All kidding aside, what a weekend! Though it didn't exactly get off to the best start…"

I patted my lap. "C'mere, *ma chère,*. You shouldn't overdo. Don't forget you were feeling sick earlier today. Just imagine, the weekend wouldn't even have happened without our first phone call. Do you remember it?"

Pittsburgh, 1995

When I left the house yesterday to participate in that golf game in Edinboro, I had no idea I'd be dreaming of my

Gettysburg dance partner tonight. So much can happen in a weekend—including golf, a barbecue, and a night with a smart, attractive woman from Erie that I could hardly leave, let alone get out of my mind.

I opened up the closet door and placed my golf clubs inside, slung my overnight bag over my shoulder and took the stairs two at a time to reach my bedroom and call Sharon. After any other overnight trip, I would unpack immediately. But not tonight. That could wait.

I snatched up the phone and sat on the edge of my king-sized bed. *What should I say?* "This is Joe." No. "Joe here. I'm back." *What if she says, Joe who? Remember the gentleman you kissed back in the Great Room? God, I'm tired. But I miss her…Guess I'll stick with "This is Joe."*

My heart beat faster, and I wiped beads of sweat off my face. With a flip of a switch, the drone of my air conditioner filled the air and blew a stream of cold air over me. *Think this through, Joe. You're freshly-divorced. She's getting a divorce. What if this is a rebound thing? What if she was just being polite?* The longer I sat there, the more doubts attacked me.

Only one way to know the answer—call her up.

She answered the phone on the first ring. "Hello."

Her voice told me how irrational I was being. I settled myself back against the headboard. "Hello, Shar, Joe here. Just got in the door."

"How was the trip back, Joe?" The warmth in her voice was unmistakable.

Should I tell her how I almost turned around three times—in Edinboro, Conneautville and Meadville—to drive back to her house and make passionate love to her? Joe, you hardly know the woman! Tell my loins that…

"*Great* drive, Shar. I was pretty much on Cloud Nine the whole way home."

I heard the sound of happy laughter, a sound I already missed. "That's good. 'Cause I was feeling the same way here."

We talked about the upcoming academic year for each of us. I lamented that our respective teaching jobs would limit our time together. "How about I come to visit you next weekend?" I held my breath.

Sharon didn't say anything for a couple of heartbeats, and I started to think the worst—*she doesn't like me. She was just being nice to me until she could get rid of me.*

Then she broke the silence. "How about I visit you?"

My heart did a happy flip-flop. I scanned the room, assessing what I'd have to do before Sharon could visit. *Could I get it done in time?* The boy in me jumped up and down, screaming: *She likes me! She likes me!*

"That'll work, too. Quick! Get something to write with. I'll give you explicit directions right to my door."

I heard her laugh again. "Joe, all I need is your address. My computer and I will do all the work. With the help of Yahoo, I'll find my way to your house."

She's telling me that she's got an independent streak and to back off! For someone like me used to tending to each detail, this caught me off guard.

All week I ran around like a little kid, making preparations for her arrival. Of course, I cleaned the house. I even vacuumed the corners and checked for cobwebs above. *What can I prepare for dinner that will knock her socks off? What about the other meals?* I pulled up a chair to the dining room table and sat down, making the first of many lists to come. After I had planned the food, I went shopping and selected the best cuts of meat, wines and other food I thought she'd like. In the days after, I devised an itinerary for sightseeing. Finally, the evening before she arrived, I mowed the grass so it would be freshly cut. I wanted everything perfect for Sharon's arrival.

As I cooked dinner that Friday night, I stole glances at the clock. *Sharon should be arriving about now.* She hadn't called to say she was leaving late, or that anything had happened. *Where can she be?*

Six o'clock passed with no sign of Sharon. I paced the carpet. At short intervals, I checked the window to scour the area for a glimpse of her car, then I went back into the kitchen.

I put the finishing touches on dinner—veal parmesan, spaghetti and a rich red sauce—setting aside the garlic bread to toast just before eating. I went to the dining room, reached into a drawer and pulled out a tablecloth with matching napkins. Back in the breakfast nook, I took two of my best dishes from the top shelf, and ran them under the faucet. After setting the silverware, I placed a wine glass at the head of each plate. I took out a couple of long candles and fished around for some crystal candlestick holders I remembered having in the drawer. I checked my watch. *It's too soon to light the candles.* I lifted the lid off the sauce and waved away the cloud of steam to take in the aroma. *Perfecto!* But for how long? I switched off the burners and wandered back into the living room.

I took a quick look around and adjusted the furniture so that each piece sat at the perfect angle. With nothing left to do, I picked up the phone and called Sharon. No one answered. *Of course, she left Erie long ago. I wish we had some way of communicating. I am sure there is some logical explanation.*

Two hours later, I teetered between anger that she had simply changed her mind and panic that something had happened to her. She could have had car trouble or an accident. God forbid, she hit a deer or some other animal. I started to pace again. Finally, I saw two headlights turn into my driveway. *She's here. Thank God, she's okay!*

I tossed the candle-lighter I'd been playing with onto the sofa and rushed down the stairs of my split-level house to open the garage door for her so she could pull her car through. I felt like I'd dropped a weight measurable not in ounces or pounds, but in *tons* at that moment.

It took all of my restraint to keep from dragging her out of the car to shower her with hugs and kisses. Instead, I managed to wait until her car came to a complete stop before bombarding her with questions about the trip. Sharon shut off the engine and popped the lock on the trunk while I saw to it the garage door closed.

Just my bad luck when I opened her door to get a kiss, she turned to grab a pie and a pan of marshmallow treats off the passenger's seat. *No kiss for me.*

"What on earth happened? I'm so glad to see you! Are you okay?"

She didn't answer. I noticed that Sharon looked disheveled and likely needed a cool drink and to relax—not a bunch of questions.

Uh-oh. This visit isn't starting out at all like I imagined it would.

She let out an audible breath. "Joe, I'm sorry I'm late. I got hopelessly lost."

"Lost? But you said—" She frowned. *Whoa. This is not an inquisition.* "Wait. Let's get you settled in. We can talk about what happened later."

Sharon wet her lips and straightened her back, as if it pained her. Then she patted her hair in place and inspected her gritty nails. "Just wondering if I could use your bathroom?"

"Oh! Sure. Of course. *Definitely.*" Suitcase and overnight bag in hand, I led her into the house. *These bags feel heavy. She plans on staying awhile. Whoo-hoo!* I couldn't help but wonder what the weekend would bring.

Just smooth this over. My hands occupied, I pointed my

chin at the finished game room. "Game room," then at the

laundry room, again, identifying it as we passed by.

Sharon led the way up the steps into the kitchen as if

she owned the place and set the pie down on the counter

along with the marshmallow treats. "It's an apple pie, you

know. Remember you told me in the great room that you

loved apple pies at this time of the year. I just threw the

other dessert together on the spur-of-the-moment."

"You did all that and teach, too? Aww." It touched me

that she took the time to bake a fancy pie like that for me.

I turned down the hall toward the master bedroom, still

carrying her luggage. "I hope you don't think I'm being too

presumptuous by putting your bags in my bedroom. I just

wanted you to have the best room in the house," I called

out over my shoulder. "Don't worry. I'm going to sleep on

the living room floor."

Sharon didn't respond though she followed me. "I need to freshen up after that long and disastrous trip."

I set her bags on the floor. I bowed deeply, took her hand and kissed it, then pointed her to the master bathroom before leaving. An amusing thought crossed my mind as I paused in the hallway. With a smile, I tapped on the door.

After a pause, "Yes?"

"Um, Sharon, I didn't get my hello kiss yet."

She didn't open the door to offer me my due. But I heard her laugh as she walked, presumably into the bathroom. The inner door clicked shut.

I walked away from the room, grinning. *At least she laughed.* We had all evening for my kiss. She came to visit me, didn't she? That meant something.

While Sharon freshened up, I opened a bottle of slightly chilled red wine and poured each of us a glass.

Then I set about to heat the rest of the food. I put the garlic toast in the oven so that it would get slightly brown. *Did my meal look classy enough? Would she think me suave and debonair?* I wanted this to be the best long-distance date she'd ever accepted.

The intoxicating scent of Shalimar drifted into the breakfast nook just ahead of Sharon as she came bouncing in. Her eyes widened at finding the round, elegant table set up there.

"Hope you don't mind, I thought it might be cozier and a little more romantic in the breakfast nook than in a ten-person formal dining room with a crystal chandelier."

Sharon gave me that wonderful accepting smile which said *it's perfect.*

I couldn't resist and bent over to plant a kiss on her neck just below her ear.

She giggled and pushed my face away. "Joe, stop! I'm

ticklish there."

"Where else are you ticklish?"

"You'll *never* find that out!" Sharon wagged a finger at me as she leaned away.

Among the clanking of silverware and tinkling of wine glasses, I learned what happened to delay Sharon earlier. "I got off the Turnpike and went onto the Parkway heading west. Then I had to go *all* the way back to the exit at Penn, um…"

"Penn Hills?"

"Yes, that's it—to turn around and ask for the directions to Monroeville. That took another two hours because I had to stop three more times to ask directions and make four U-turns." She took a sip of wine and let it wash down before she spoke again. "But here I am, safe and sound."

"That's right. Is it any wonder it wasn't worse? If you

had only allowed me to give you directions, I could have gotten you right to my doorstep."

She raised an eyebrow. "I made it here, didn't I?"

"You certainly did." I took her hand to let her know how happy her being here made me. I rather liked how she had the stamina to keep searching until she found my house, except, of course, that she scared the hell out of me. "More wine?"

She nodded and I topped her glass. "Joe, the veal and spaghetti are delicious. You are quite the chef." She licked her fingers after finishing off a thick slice of toasted garlic bread. "I'll have another, if that's okay."

Things are definitely looking up now.

Afterward, Sharon helped me clear off the table and do the dishes. As we cleaned up, I explained the various options I'd looked into for our sightseeing tour. "Okay, where would you like to go first?"

"Surprise me."

I emptied out the dishpan and pulled the plug in the sink, letting the water gurgle down the drain. "Okay, I know what we'll do. We can do *quid pro quo* with me taking you on tours here in Pittsburgh and you showing me the sights in Erie. How about that?"

"It's a deal." Dish towel in hand, Sharon looked right at home. I felt as if I'd known her longer than two—no, three—dates if I counted the first time we danced together at Gettysburg College as a date. It really wasn't, but I liked thinking of it as one. This was the first time I'd ever agreed to a long-term dating relationship. It felt pretty damn good.

As we finished the dishes, Sharon reached over the edge of the counter to hang up the dish towel. At the same time, I bent over to put away a large saucepan. We bumped heads.

"Oh, sorry." Sharon rubbed my forehead where she

banged into it.

"No problem. I shouldn't have—"

She giggled. I laughed. Our nervousness made me realize that our feelings were moving too fast and in a dangerous direction. Sharon looked into my eyes and then looked away. I knew what my heart was urging me to do.

Yet, it wasn't the right time. Or was it?

I led Sharon down the hallway and into my bedroom. We both sat on the king-size bed. The same bed that my ex-wife slept in for the better part of twenty years while I, many times, sought refuge in the family room. We hadn't been happily intimate for years, not since we drifted apart.

No. We can't do this. Instead of holding and kissing Shar as I imagined just moments ago, I sat on the bed with my elbows on my knees and my head in my hands. Sharon rubbed my back. "Are you feeling all right?"

"Shar, the timing isn't right, if you know what I mean.

The emotional turmoil alone from our past marriages is making us more vulnerable. You're still getting over all the crap your ex did to you. I don't want us to jump into anything. What we're feeling are natural urges but...."

She looked at me. *Was that disappointment?* "You're right." She didn't say anything for a little bit. "You're right. Yes." She sighed deeply. It was clear she was fighting the same urges I was. She sat a little further from me. "And you know ... I have a thing about God. He wouldn't ... couldn't ... bless it."

"Let's just see what God is going to do in our relationship," she said.

I cleared my throat. "In the meantime, we'll get to know each other a little better. Our families and friends will get a better sense of who we are..."

"Joe, we're making the right decision to wait. I'm glad we talked it through instead of giving in to our desires."

"Now, if I could only convince my body of that." I leaned in and hugged her. "Ohhh," I groaned as she ran her fingers through my hair. Tilting my face up, I kissed her with feeling. *Stop that.* I stood up, took her shoulders in my hand and kissed her cheek like a grandfather might do. "Good night, Sunshine. Pleasant dreams," I said leaving the room.

Making my way to the family room with my pillow, blanket and pajamas in my arms, I couldn't get the scent of her perfume out of my head. I couldn't fit on the sofa without my feet sticking up in the air so the floor would have to do. Though carpeted, it felt very hard and painful. As I lay near the cold fireplace, I tried to ease myself into a comfortable position. I hadn't felt at all like a grandfather —until now with all these aches and pains. I folded over my pillow and sank back into it. *Was she asleep? Was she thinking of me right now? I wish I were by her side. No, you don't. Remember the decision we just made. Go to sleep.*

I rolled onto my side and slammed my head against the log carrier, letting loose a string of curse words. I rubbed my head where I found a raw welt. I grabbed a couple of lounge pillows and stuck them behind my head, switched on the TV and immersed myself in some late night movies. Eventually, I fell asleep, my arms wrapped around a bed pillow and my head lolling backward against the couch.

Fully awake the next morning, I tried not to think of Sharon sleeping in the master bedroom a few steps away. I tiptoed down the hallway to the bathroom, trying not to wake Sleeping Beauty. I left the bathroom and paused at the door. No noise.

"Are you awake?" I whispered.

When I didn't get an answer, I pushed the door open a crack and saw Sharon covered from her toes to her nose, her hair splayed over the pillow. Her own pillow she brought from Erie. She'd said, "It's like an American Express card. I never leave home without it."

She looked so peaceful lying there that I nearly backed out of the room and closed the door behind me. But I couldn't resist leaning over to say, "Good morning, Sunshine."

I heard a muffled, "What time is it?"

"Seven o'clock."

"You're a good guy, Joe. But it's a little early, don't you think?"

"Maybe." I didn't want to tell her this was right on time for me. How nice it would be to wake up next to her and say "Good morning, Sunshine" every time we woke up. She closed her eyes and fell back asleep. I lay on the covers, my hands behind my head, thinking. I'm a good guy? Last night was a testament to both of us being good guys, behaving ourselves.

In my heart, I was hoping that God would hurry up and give us a sign. Then again, I knew He had His own timetable. My being in a rush would have no bearing on when He'd work out the details.

Sharon cuddled up to me on the sofa, her head on my chest as I finished our walk down memory lane. "We finally got the timing right," I said.

"*Merci beaucou*p. *Je t'adore mon amour.*"

"Wait a minute. 'Mercy buckets' to you, too. No fair. You actually *speak* French."

"I speak Spanish and some Italian, too: *Marco Polo.*" She snickered.

"Marco Polo? Are you trying to pull the wool over my eyes? … so what's your point?"

"…that you'd prepare a fantastic Thanksgiving dinner this year, *monsieur* top chef.

"I beg to differ. How could you forget the dismal failure I met up with during our first Thanksgiving meal together?"

Sharon smacked my hand. "Oh honey, it wasn't a failure!"

"It flopped, like a bad pancake."

"It did *not!* We just grew up with different traditions and tastes."

"I'll say…"

***

Erie, 1995

What a joyous occasion. I had so much to be thankful for. My ex-wife had moved out and was enjoying her new life in Albuquerque. My life was starting to fall together nicely. This holiday, I found myself in Erie, Summit

Township, really, and would soon meet Sharon's mom, her sister, Paula, and brother-in-law, Gregg.

I can't wait to show off my talents as a better-than-average cook!

Sharon would provide the main meal, and her family, the side dishes. For starters, Sharon would roast the turkey, make stuffing and gravy. She'd already baked several pies for dessert. Everyone in the family contributed some dish, even Sharon's sons. To my surprise, Stuart planned to bring a delicious apple crisp and two potato dishes. Mrs. Starks, Sharon's mother, would bring her signature potato dumplings.

A couple days before Thanksgiving, I took a few minutes out from grading hundreds of student exams to let Sharon know what I planned to bring. "I'll make soup, a hot veggie dish, and one of my delicious potato specialties. Is that all right?"

"Sure. Your son Jason, is he coming?"

"Not too thrilled about it but hopefully, he'll get to know Matt and Stuart a little better."

"Good. Gotta go now. I'm marking exams. See you Thursday morning."

We arrived early; refrigerating the dishes I'd brought until we could warm them up for our early dinner. My son Jason joined Matt and Stuart and some of the others in the living room as I helped Sharon get ready. Finally, I set the table and we invited everyone to sit down.

When we served the meal, the wheels fell off our smooth-running Thanksgiving Express.

Our first mistake, we served dinner a la Belan, in set courses. The empty crockery awaited the piping hot, homemade vegetable-turkey soup, which sat smack in the middle of the table. The guests looked from person to person, as if to say, "What's next?" I ladled one scoop of soup into each bowl. Sharon's family looked at me, down at the bowl and back to me again. Not a single one of them touched the soup. They didn't seem to pick up on the hint the turkey vegetable soup was the first course.

When I finished eating my lonely little bowl of soup, the next course came out—the salad. I kept saying, "Dig in!" and "Help yourself," but only half the family did. The main meal came next. As if starving, the families enthusiastically pounced on the food, passing it around the table every which way. Everything disappeared during that meal with the exception of the turkey soup, the mushrooms and my potato dumplings.

After Sharon and I cleared the table, we started on the dishes. I kissed her. "Fabulous dinner, honey. But I got a question. Can you enlighten me? I thought I would impress your family with my culinary skills. But the soup bombed. My delicious sautéed buttered mushrooms fared no better.

And my poor little potato dumplings got ignored." I shook my head in comic bewilderment.

"Well—" Sharon giggled.

"Even my beautiful girlfriend, if that's who she really is and not an alien invading her body, ate just enough to get by."

She put a hand on her hip and shook a finger at me. "I was trying to be diplomatic and that's not an easy task, I'll have you know."

"Diplomatic. Now you are in the Diplomatic Corps? Whoa. Is this a war between the Belans and the Starks?" I teased.

She bit her lip and tried not to laugh. "I'm sorry, Joe." She fanned herself with a cloth napkin. "The thing is my family just heaps up all the food on the table at once, and that's ... uh, how we ... eat. We're a pretty informal family when all is said and done."

"I see noooow." I laughed. "The exact opposite of my family. I grew up eating a formal, multi-course Thanksgiving dinner. Each course had distinct tableware, which my mother collected after we ate it. Then she dispensed new tableware for the next course. It started out with the soup, followed by a salad. Then we had turkey and the trimmings, and, of course, finished with dessert. But we had one more tradition: everyone in the Belan household would rub their full bellies and drink a small liqueur aperitif at the end of the meal."

"Oh my. From the way you talked, I got the idea your family made a big to-do out of the holiday. I thought my family would rise to the occasion. No such luck."

I shook my head I mock dismay. "But even if we eat differently, why didn't they at least *try* my food?"

"The thing is we don't have any soup eaters on our side. I feel bad but I guess I should tell you that no one in the family likes mushrooms either."

"Well, they certainly seemed to like the *potatoes*. Why didn't they try them?" Though I put on a show of huffing and puffing my displeasure, she knew I didn't mean it, too much, anyway.

"I don't know. I guess they thought it was disrespectful to eat your dumplings and not eat Grandma Stark's special dumplings. *I* ate a few, though and they tasted delicious."

"Well, thank God, you and Jason both did." I sniffed and wiped away my fake tears.

"I'm so sorry. Joe, I didn't know exactly what you were making ahead of time so I couldn't give you a head's up. Then, when I found out this morning, it got awkward. I didn't know how to tell you that you chose the worst possible dishes. Are you upset?"

"Nah. But if you'd just told me..." I stooped over and scraped just above the floor with a spatula, made a show of folding an imaginary object and of sliding it in my back pocket.

As Sharon watched me, her eyes got wide. "What are you doing?"

"Just scraping up my ego off the floor and saving it for later."

"Oh, you!"

We had a laugh, but I still had to visit with her family and carry on as if nothing had happened. Our first Thanksgiving meal together demanded as much. But I had learned my lesson. The next time, I made just enough soup for me -- only to find the tureen empty by the time it got around to me. *Go figure.*

"So you see, Sunshine, while I was trying to prove that I was better-than-average cook and make favorable first impressions, it backfired."

"No way, honey. You're a culinary marvel." Sharon

protested. "My family didn't know what they were missing that meal. Besides that, they laughed and laughed when you told your funny stories." She covered my face in little kisses. "Won't you puh-leaze make dinner this year?"

"Well, I'd never turn down a pretty wife like you. I'll have to make up a list…"

We'd make it through Thanksgiving. But what would Christmas and New Year's bring? *Joe, one day at a time. She made it through the surgery. She's recovering. Soon your life will be back on an even keel.*

Chapter 7
CHRISTMAS AND ICE DUNES

December rolled in, white and cold. Sharon insisted on preparing for this holiday exactly as we would any other one. So, we started decorating the house right after Thanksgiving. Then came the baking.

"Hang on, before you dash into pie-baking mode, think about it. Just a few weeks ago, your health was up in the air. We were debating even cooking Thanksgiving dinner. Now you're all gung-ho on making God-knows-how-many pies. Does that make sense to you?"

Sharon sat at a table, browsing through several recipes. "It's what I do best. The 'funnest' part of preparing for any holiday."

I sighed. She wasn't getting it. "This is serious, Shar. When I think of all the emergencies we went through—it's not a debate of wills. It's your *health*."

All three of 'our' sons had come to stay and were hanging out in the living room. Stuart, Sharon's oldest, was leafing through the newspaper, and Matt and Jason had launched into a debate on the best places to see in Pittsburgh.

"Thank you for your concern, but really I'm fine now." She faced the boys, "What kind of pies shall I make for Christmas this year?"

The requests ranged from apple to lemon meringue— five in all. I waited to see how it would play out. The family had to be reasonable. She couldn't please them all, could she?

She glanced my way. "Don't worry. Come Christmas Day, there'll be each of their favorite pies waiting for them." My jaw dropped down. "I'll make them this week and freeze them for the holiday. You see, I won't be rushed and everyone will be happy."

I put my foot down. "Only if you let me help you."

"Okay. Just this one time."

She dictated a list to me and we shopped for all the ingredients she needed. The next morning, she donned a festive apron and got to work. She kicked everyone but me out of the kitchen. A good thing I stayed. In the course of her baking, open containers, mixing tools, egg shells, apple peelings all littered the table, counter tops, and stove. I ran around picking up discarded utensils, washing them and placing them within her reach before she could miss them —or so I tried, anyway.

A buzzer went off. Shar turned in a circle, a smudge of flour on her face and the string of her apron trailing near her feet. "Where is my sifter? Joe, I can't find my measuring spoons. What did you do with them?"

"One question at a time," I said, already looking for

the lost items.

"Joe, I have a system and you're moving things."

"It's not going to do you any good to have dirty utensils lying around…" I began reasonably. "I'm merely *helping* you."

"Well, *don't!* You're invading my space." She finally found the sifter and pointed it at me. "Thank you but that's enough. I'll work faster if you leave me alone!"

"I couldn't let you …"

"You're getting in the way. Honey, I know you mean well, but please…"

"I'm not doing anything. If you keep a neat kitchen—"

"Joe, get out!" Hands folded across her chest, she glared daggers.

Never had she looked cuter than at that moment, with a dusting of flour on her cheek and a daub of butter on her arm. I gave her a quick peck on the forehead and ducked out, laughing. "I suppose it's too late to put in an order for minced meat pie," I called, ready to dodge in the event she threw a rolling pin my way.

"Out!"

That night as we snuggled under the covers, she said, "Okay, we can cross the pies off our list. Ummm … there's only one thing..." She had that serious look on her face.

"What's that?" I frowned as her cold toes met my feet. I covered them with my much larger ones. The sooner she warmed up, the more comfortable I'd feel.

"Joe, I know you mean well. But I'm recovering from the cancer now. I know you want to help me, but it doesn't work with you in the kitchen. How about if we make a rule? When I cook, you stay out. And when you cook, I stay out?"

"I don't mind you being there," I drew her close and nibbled on her ear.

"Stop, that tickles." She wiggled away and tried to be diplomatic. "Well, I *do* mind you being there. To be honest, your neatness drives me up the wall."

I pulled away. I'd really only been trying to help. Her way, it would take hours to clean up after. As it was, she looked exhausted after her day of baking. "I'm just wired that way. If I know a better way, why can't I—" *No. That line of reasoning didn't work in my other relationships. It wouldn't fly here either.* In a conciliatory tone, I finally said, "If that's what you want, I'll stay out." *I'll respect her wishes and if that means giving her space in the kitchen to do her thing, by God, I'll do it.*

"Thanks, sweetheart." She turned on her side and put an arm around my waist. "Now we need to start our Christmas shopping."

"Yeah, cuddle up and drop the next bomb."

***

One week after Thanksgiving, I said, "Let the madness begin." We made lists (my idea) and set out Christmas shopping after Sharon left work one day. We hurried through the department stores, bypassing the fake Santa Clauses and their ho-ho-hos, and past the decorated storefronts with their red *SALE!* tags on the display mannequins and electronic goods. We lingered longingly as the sweet aromas of cinnamon, chocolate mint mocha and peppermint mingled together by ice cream and coffee shops.

The crowds of people surged forward en masse like huge barges expecting us, like so many smaller watercraft, to clear out of their pathways in the aisle ahead. I knew Sharon had reached her limit when she slumped on a bench and steadied a trembling leg with her hand.

I sat down next to her. "Are you all right?"

"Joe, it's a little too much during the week after a full day of teaching. So many people … they just shove you out of the way and they cough without covering their mouths."

Yeah, and they probably didn't wash their hands after going to the bathroom either.

Sharon must stay safe. I need to get her out of this germ-exposed area. But I don't want to seem like a mother hen. On the other hand, I want her well enough to enjoy the holiday. A cold could kill her with her weakened system.

"If we go again, it'll have to be on a weekend. It's doesn't make sense but fewer people go out then." I brushed her hair out of her eyes and held her shaking body close to mine.

"Where's the list?" she asked.

I took it out of my wallet and presented it to her. With a quick once-over she sighed. "We will have to go again.

We have a lot of the grandkids to buy for yet."

"Are you hungry?

"Starved. You know, I remember going Christmas shopping with my mom a long time ago. We'd go the *Boston Store*. It was six floors, and very nice. We'd split up and she'd say 'Meet me under the clock at three o'clock' or some such time. We usually had a bite to eat at a cafeteria in the basement, which sold bargain goods. But one time after meeting up, we got to go into this upscale restaurant, for that time period anyway, and eat soup and hot tea. I loved it. It was just my mom and I that day."

"They have a really nice pub under the clock now," I observed, contemplating taking Sharon there for old time's sake.

"Yes … I remember you could enter the store from three different locations—Peach Street, State Street and Eighth Street. I loved that place…"

"Well, do you fancy going there now? Think about it while I get the car. I'll pick you right up at the mall entrance. We'll get caught in the Peach Street jam anyway. We'll have time to decide. Are you sure you'll be all right?"

Though she nodded, I exited the mall as fast as I could. She didn't look good. Come to think of it, maybe it would be better to get her home so she could relax. I made a mental note to take her there when she felt better.

With a few days' rest, Sharon bounced back. We spent the remaining weekends shopping at discount outlet stores. As we neared the double glass doors in front, the *ding-ding-ding* of a lone bell ringer bracing against the cold wind always caught Sharon's eye, and she dropped a few dollar bills into the red kettle. "God bless you," the volunteer said each time and commenced ringing the bell once more.

As we left the pepperoni warmth of *Patti's Pizza* and

stepped into the cold again, I reached for Sharon's gloved hand. "I'm stuffed, aren't you?" I patted my belly with my free hand. "Shar, I still have the dilemma of deciding what to buy you this year. C'mon, give me a clue here."

"The last time you asked me that question, you regretted it—at least in the beginning," she teased.

"Did I ever. I call that "the Koinonia Extortion." I pretended to push her away from me but made sure not to knock her over. The wind whistled through the barren trees as we continued to make our way to the car.

Sharon paused to pull up a fallen sock inside her boot. "Has that only been a couple of years now?"

"Yes, that's right. You bribed me two years after we got married." I shook a finger at her as I waited for her to fix her other sock, which had also fallen down in her boot.

"Joe, do you really call it that?" She sounded shocked.

"I sure do. Let me refresh your memory."

***

Erie, Late Autumn 2001

Ever since we met, Sharon and I had exchanged

meaningful and somewhat expensive Christmas gifts, like

leather coats and pricy jewels, as Sharon called them, for

her. She'd buy me nice brand watches like Swiss or Cartier

and top-of-the-line sweaters. But this time, I ran into a

brick wall when it came to choosing the right gifts.

I tried a number of covert tactics to determine what she

would like. When we shopped for jewelry, I would steal

glances her way to see if any put a sparkle in her eye, and

maybe a clue. I observed as we traipsed in and out of

stores. But nothing. I hinted around about specialty items,

by saying "Did you see the scarf that Mary had? Wouldn't

you look good wearing that?" I even checked out the hall

closet thinking that maybe a nice fur coat would fill the bill.

But Sharon didn't seem to go for any kind of fur. Nothing seemed to work. Finally, I just blurted out, "I'm stumped, Shar. Give me a hint what to buy you." I got nothing from her in the way of a suggestion.

Then one day as we sat in the living room watching *It's a Wonderful Life* with Jimmy Stewart and Donna Reed, she raised the subject. "Do you really want to know what I'd like as a Christmas present from you?"

Now we were making headway. I leaned forward, "I will give you anything your heart desires."

"Anything?

"Anything." My beautiful wife deserved the very best. I didn't care about the cost. I just wanted to make her happy. 'You want the moon? Just say the word and I'll throw a lasso around it and pull it down for you,'" I said, in my best Jimmy Stewart imitation.

"Clever, very clever. Do you remember the part where

George Bailey and his wife, Mary, are dancing the Charleston and they fall into a pool?"

I laughed. "How's your Charleston?"

Sharon got up off the sofa and spun around, facing me. She snapped her fingers and did a fair rendition of the dance, kicking her feet up. She stopped and collapsed on the sofa, laughing.

"Not bad at all. Okay, so back to my question, you were going to tell me what I could get you."

"Oh, yes." She put her arm on one shoulder, and drew me to her. I noticed she had a big cat-that-ate-the-canary grin on her face. "I want you to go to Koinonia. "

I slumped down on the sofa, "Aww, Shar. Not the men's religious retreat. That's a whole weekend."

Her lips fell into a pout. "You said, 'Anything.'"

I took the pen she offered and signed the application form that magically appeared in her hands.

Somewhere in the back of my mind, a Bible story came to me. "Was it some king—King Herod, maybe—who made an oath to some beautiful maiden who danced for him." I looked pointedly at my wife and grinned, warming to my story. "King Herod said to the girl, 'Ask *me for anything you want, and you shall have it.*'"

"*Ooooh. You're talking about Queen Herodias's daughter, and John the Baptist.*" Sharon covered her mouth with her hands. "*Are you comparing me to the dancer, or worse, that evil queen?*" She pretended to be shocked. "*You are so naughty!*"

"*Anyway, the girl…*"

She shook a finger at me. "*His daughter, Salome.*"

"*… requested that he behead John the Baptist and serve it on a platter. Since King Herod had made a vow, he had to follow through with her wishes even though it worried him.*"

Sharon put her hands on her hips, and her jaw dropped down. "What? Do you think Koinonia is something terrible like that? Are you worried now? "

"Nah, of course not." Even though going on the retreat was the last thing I wanted to do, I'd made a promise to the woman—my wife—and I meant to keep that promise.

"Besides," she said, "There is a long waiting list and you might not even be selected to go. Even then, you'll still have the option to decline."

Yeah, like you're going to let that happen.

Luck was not with me. The selection process didn't take long at all. I had to "report for duty" one Friday night in mid-November. Fortunately, it took place on a weekend that the Steelers had an away game.

The weekend turned out to be the most dynamic, life-altering weekend of my life. When I was given my cross on Sunday, I cried. I felt almost as happy as the day that

Sharon and I got married.

"So your tricking me into going actually turned out to be something pretty great," I remarked

The television caught our attention again. *George Bailey leaned over to Mary and whispered softly*, 'You're wonderful, just wonderful.'

"Aw, that's such a sweet scene." Sharon muted the volume and crossed her arms in a challenge. "Well, at least I did something right. I knew you'd like it if you only gave the men's retreat a chance. "

"I reconnected to God and learned the importance of prayer all over again. Along the way we sang a lot."

"However it came about, I'm glad it did." Sharon cozied up to me and we started dancing around the living room and down the hallway. One thing led to another, and before we knew it, we'd closed the bedroom door behind us.

Lying under the covers later, I sat up and looked at her. "You never answered me. What very special gift should I buy you this year?"

"Honey, I'm so thankful to be here at all. Please don't buy me anything. I don't want material things. I just want to celebrate my life and the success of my operation. Anything else would cheapen this gift, do you know what I mean?"

"Aww, but Shar—"

"I'm serious. You can buy me one small object this year. That's it."

I mulled it over for a couple of days. What would mean something to her? It needs to be symbolic. Nothing seemed quite right. Finally, it came to me what I could buy her. I felt kind of silly. *It's so little. Will she get it?*

On Christmas morning as I lay in bed waiting for Sharon to wake up, I could hardly contain my excitement.

I'm like a little boy! Unable to stay in bed any longer, I got up and made some coffee. I was just pouring a cup and waiting for the toast to pop up when Sharon walked into the kitchen. "Good morning, Sunshine."

"Mornin' Joe. Merry Christmas." That's when I got my Christmas 'mornin' kiss.

As soon as we'd eaten and cleaned up the kitchen, I retrieved the gift—all wrapped up with a big fancy bow on it—and handed it to her.

"Honey, since we are exchanging gifts, let me go get yours." She went into our bedroom. I heard the closet door open and close. She returned with a package and handed it to me.

I gently pushed her onto the sofa. "Open yours first."

She eased the bow off and with the tip of her nail, undid the tape. She gave me a questioning look and slid the box out of the wrapping. "An electric pencil sharpener. Joe, this is so cool! I have just the place for it in my classroom. It's perfect! I'm going to be teaching for a long time yet..."

I smiled and opened my own gift. "Oh Shar, golf balls —and a wrist brace. Just what I need to stop my golf slice." I chuckled. "Perfect gifts for a year in which we are grateful for our lives above anything else."

***

New Year's Eve was a quiet affair. We watched the ball drop with Dick Clark on television. We clinked glasses of champagne together as we sipped it. But halfway through, we left the glasses and made beautiful love just after midnight.

***

As Erie winds whipped the weather into an icy frenzy soon after the New Year, I talked Sharon into going to Presque Isle. Although the cold didn't hamper me, it made Sharon shudder. The first sign of those white, ice crystals gently drifting from the sky would send me into a frenzy of excitement, so she indulged me every now and again.

"This will give you the perfect opportunity to scout out those craggly trees you like so much," I said. Sharon loved to search out the most barren outgrowths and photograph them against the sky. She would take hundreds of photographs, and not only of trees but desolate grass, clouds, skylines and every possible nuance of sky color. She'd then study the photographs. Eventually, they'd wind up in a composite landscape she'd paint. She focused on landscapes in her paintings. She'd include all the elements that inspired her.

Painting was more than a hobby for Sharon. It

incorporated her observations, her artistic skills and her faith in one ongoing messy package. Painting was a lifestyle form of art for her, like an ongoing dialogue with nature.

She'd involve me and ask my opinion of this cloud or that light. "I'm not qualified to give my opinion," I'd protest. She wasn't happy unless she got some response. So I began to look at these things and try to be more knowledgeable, too. She invited me into her world of artistic design, an integral part of who she was. No one had ever done that with me before.

This year we drove for quite awhile, pulling over to allow Sharon the chance to take her photos. We then continued on our way. I loved seeing Presque Isle at its most natural form—dazzling white. I recalled the first time I ever saw the ice dunes in Erie, nearly eight years ago.

Erie, 1995

"I have something marvelous to show you," Sharon said one weekend. "Erie has a lot of beautiful sights to see, and Presque Isle in winter is definitely one of the best."

We got in the car and drove. Once we arrived in the park, she said, "Pull over."

"Where? Here?" I parked the car in a little indent off the road. Sharon covered my eyes for a moment. The wool from her thick finger-mittens scratched my eyelids.

"Are you ready?"

"I am."

"You're not going to believe your eyes," she said. "Look around."

As I opened my eyes, I saw what looked like six to ten feet high waves breaking on the shore, except that the waves were frozen. It looked like time had just stopped in mid-motion. *So these were ice dunes. Incredibly beautiful.* "Pittsburgh doesn't have anything this spectacular." I breathed.

"Yep, gorgeous. But did you read the signs? You have to be very careful." The signs warned in big black letters: DANGER: KEEP OFF THE ICE DUNES.

"The danger comes when people climb and walk on the dunes. They're quite deceptive. The thing is that they're hollow underneath. If someone falls through an ice dune, they'll get caught inside a hollow cave half-filled with icy water. Not only does hypothermia set in, it's really dangerous for others to rescue them." She shuddered.

Sharon and I wisely kept our distance. I took out my camera and snapped some excellent photos to show people back home. "If I'd have known how beautiful Erie was, I'd have tried to meet you a long time ago. I've known you less than six months but it's been the best six months of my life."

"You really loved those ice dunes, didn't you?" Sharon

exclaimed, leaning up against a spiny, withered tree. She balanced her foot on a weathered, forlorn looking picnic table and clicked a dozen more photographs. She chuckled and shook her head. "I enjoyed showing you the sites in Erie whatever the season. You were so easy to impress."

"I must have been under your spell that year. And every year since."

"You're so funny. I dazzled you straight off with the ice dunes, but it took me quite awhile to get you to appreciate all the beautiful clouds in the sky. C'mon, let's get some pictures. Look at that ice dune over there." I looked over to where she pointed. "2004 is a good year for ice dunes, you know."

The cold kept us indoors much of the winter. Sharon couldn't tolerate Erie's freezing temperatures very well. But we didn't mind. We'd watch TV or read books on weekends. We thrived on the debate that surrounded them

—well, most of the time. One afternoon as we stretched out on the sofa watching a detective movie on the boob tube, Sharon said, "Look at that! That wouldn't happen in real life. It's so contrived."

Almost dozing, I opened one eye. "Huh?"

She jabbed me. "Wake up. Pay attention. This plot has so many holes in it. I can't believe it actually passed muster. Who selected this made-for-TV movie anyway?"

That was my cue. I was expected to *say* something. "There you go. Obviously the producer has underestimated the intelligence of the average Saturday afternoon viewer." I yawned.

"You have no idea what I'm talking about here, do you? Are you even watching this?"

"Have a heart. Just on the verge of sleep here…" I protested.

"Well, go back to Snoresville. I'll have this debate with

someone else."

For the record, she continued to debate me though I didn't have much to contribute on the believability of this particular movie. I threw in a few half-hearted attempts at both agreeing and disagreeing with her. But she saw through my real lack of interest and griped, "If you don't really care, I'd rather you just take a nap." She liked a good debate.

"Next time, Shar…I owe you one. Here, why not take a nap with me. It's a God-awful movie with bad dialogue anyway…"

We also debated over the plots of our favorite contemporary authors—Stephen King, John Sanford, Nelson DeMille or Sandra Brown—along with literary works, and radio talk shows. We compared authors and discussed evolving styles. Verbally sparring with Shar made me feel like I had my wife back. I welcomed these little normalities with great fervor, except, of course, when

I was half asleep. And that spoke volumes all by itself. It

meant I didn't have to hold on to every word Sharon said,

as if it were our last. *Life felt good.*

Chapter 8
IN REMISSION

Sharon was in remission. Slowly, we started to relax and let go of the fear we'd been steeped in the past several months. Fully engrossed in her teaching, Sharon now carried the problems of her kids on her shoulders and let go of her own. She had a wonderful rapport with her co-workers and often shared stories of their support.

One day she bounced into the house all excited, sweeping me up in a kiss. "Thank you for the beautiful bouquet of flowers you had sent to my classroom, Joe. The kids teased me about 'my boyfriend' all afternoon." She looked like a schoolgirl herself the way she was blushing. "The other teachers got sooo jealous."

"I'll have to remember to send them more often."

"One teacher said, "It must be nice when you're so

sick to have a husband who sends you flowers.' Is that a backhanded compliment or what?" She giggled nervously. "I don't know. They still think I'm sick even though I've been back to work for several months now."

"Honey, I don't think she meant anything by it. Poor lady probably never received any flowers at her home let alone her workplace. Shall I send her some, too?"

"I don't think so." She gave me a stern look meant to put me in my place. "I told her that you just liked to send me flowers. For no reason at all."

"And because *you* like it," I reminded.

She gave me a small smile. "Hon, why am I so sensitive about being called 'sick?' It's so silly. My co-workers always look after me. But anyway, I'm so ready to move on."

"Knock on wood."

"My kiddies kept crowding around my desk to touch

the petals and 'ooh,' over the roses, even the boys. You know, little Paul? He said he wanted to send me 'bunches of flowers till my desk overflowed' because 'you're my favorite teacher in the world.' Isn't that adorable? He was a little worried you'd get mad at him though."

"Mad? Why would I get mad?"

"The competition."

I laughed. "Pretty ladies always have competition. I might have an edge, though."

"I don't know. Paul is pretty darn cute. He knows just what to say to get on my good side…"

I'm glad I made it a habit to send flowers to Sharon at work. This is one of the most positive suggestions that came out of our couple's counseling.

Although we had a good relationship, Sharon wanted to avoid any pitfalls or past mistakes so she talked me into going to counseling. This turned out to be the best thing we could do for our marriage. It all started with The Funeral—that's how we always refer to it. We both know immediately which one.

Erie, 1998

Sharon and I always supported each other. At times, she had to deal in public with her ex in ways that infuriated her. The funeral of their mutual friend brought them together once more—understandable up to a point. But Sharon's ex used the occasion as a chance to flaunt his mistress-turned-spouse.

The couple stood, arm-in-arm, peering down into the casket. A few minutes later, they moved to talk to some friends. Through it all, the woman rained small kisses on his good-for-nothing shoulder as they held hands or otherwise caressed each other.

"Look at them, all lovely-dovey." Sharon stood, transfixed, her small chest heaving in and out. "How *dare* he come here and behave like that!"

"Ahhh, Shar, ignore them." I wanted to go and beat the guy up.

Her nostrils flared and her eyes burned holes into their backs but she didn't say anything. I pointed to the guest book in hopes of distracting her. "Sharon, let's sign in."

She grabbed the pen and jabbed it down the list. She found what she was looking for—their names. I didn't know what to think. I'd never seen Sharon so put-out. *She's not going to cross out their names, is she?* I sighed in relief as she scrawled her name and handed me the pen. Yet part of me had wanted to goad her on. *You go, girl. Cross 'em out. Add some graffiti if it makes you feel better.* She squared her shoulders. "Shall we give our condolences?"

Sharon extended all the courtesies that one would expect of her on such a somber occasion. She murmured words of encouragement and embraced grieving family members and friends. Probably no one else even noticed anything amiss. But after nearly four years with her, I could read her body language well. She stood like a chiseled statue, folding her arms across her chest. Every once in awhile, I'd see her eyes narrow and scan the room. As her ex and his wife made their way around the place, she always seemed to know where to find them.

As we drove home, the mood turned as dark as the night around us.

"He had the nerve to show up—with *her!*" Sharon said through gritted teeth. "I *knew* he'd come. I could just….wring…his…neck."

"Shar, think about it. Didn't you take a good look at her? She has *nothing* on you. There is no accounting for tastes. Of course, he shouldn't have brought her—or even come himself."

My wife cheated on me. *I know that feeling of*

betrayal. But at least the guy she cheated with didn't live around the corner from me. I never had to see the two of them together or hear about their latest indiscretion from the neighbors. *That's enough to kill you right there.*

"Did you see how every man envied me? You looked absolutely stunning."

"Oh, Joe, nobody looks stunning at a funeral." She let one hand rest on my leg. I glanced down at her plain slender fingers and the clear polished nails. I wouldn't mind seeing my wedding ring on her finger. *One day.*

I nudged her with my leg. "You did, I'm serious. Much more vibrant and full of life than say…the dead lady in the box."

"Joe!" She smoothed out the fabric of my suit. "Actually, the mortuary did a good job with her, don't you think?"

I'd never really been a fan of the make-up that

mortuaries put on dead people. They aren't going anywhere, are they? I rolled my eyes but managed to keep a straight face. "Mmm. But the service seemed a little too formal. I almost fell asleep and you know me when I sleep…"

"Thank *God*, you didn't. Can you imagine?" She gave her rendition of my snore, ending in several small snorts. "Your snores would interrupt the reverend's eulogy. On cue, everyone would turn around and stare. And there would be *no* envy element involved."

"I beg your pardon. Are you suggesting there would be pity for you?"

"That just might be the case." I took my hand off the wheel for a moment and squeezed hers. The mood was lifting.

But later on that night, I found her in the living room, her Bible nearby with a crumpled tissue in the fold. Sharon sat forward, gripping the arm of the tan leather sofa. Tears coursed down her face. "I did everything I could to be a good wife, kept a good house, had a steady job, took good care of the boys, got involved in their classes at school. Why wasn't it good enough for him, Joe?"

"He was a jerk, that's why. He didn't appreciate what he had."

She clutched several soggy tissues. "I deserved better, didn't I?" Her voice was muffled. She tapped her fingers against her lips again and again.

She was making me nervous. I took her hands and stilled them between my own. "Shar, look, if he hadn't been so selfish, I wouldn't be in this room with you now, right?"

It was as if I hadn't spoken. Some days, she'd hold onto my every word. Not tonight. Though her divorce came through a couple of months after we started dating, nearly four years later, she still struggled, on occasion, with guilt and insecurity.

I had to make her see… "Honey, it wasn't up to you. One person can't make a marriage work. He left you. You got divorced legally, and went through the church to have your marriage annulled. It's kosher in the eyes of the church and even God himself."

"I just *hate* it. Maybe if I had been better at…"

Kneeling down on the carpet in front of her, I tried to still her trembling body. "Shar, look, even your legs are shaking. It's not worth all this emotion." I took her in my arms awkwardly. "Shar, you didn't need to be any better."

I cursed under my breath. Part of me wanted to grab her and knock some sense into that head of hers. But another part just wanted make up for the stunts he pulled and reassure her.

She stiffened in my arms. *Uh-oh.* This called for

drastic measures. I had an idea.

"Shar, what can I do make you stop crying? Do you want the dog in me to come out?" I began to crawl around the floor, barking. The sight of my bulky frame moving around on all fours brought the hoped-for peels of laughter. "You're insane. Joe, I'm going through a crisis. This is no time to joke around. Okay, okay, I'll stop."

I cradled her in my arms as we laughed. *Crisis averted.*

In bed and cuddled up close, I broached the subject. "Sharon, I know you're seeing that counselor. Is he still helping you?"

"Honey, go with me."

"Forget it. I have no faith in them after dealing with that jackass, crappy counselor at my son's school!" I had my fill of other school counselors throughout my career, too. "Pencil pushers and paper shufflers, the lot of 'em."

"Joe, just go with me once. This counselor is different.

If you don't like him, I won't make you go back, I promise. He's actually helped me a lot."

Trying to save her marriage, she'd said when she mentioned seeing the counselor at first. Only her ex stopped going with her after the first couple of times. She continued going alone. After their divorce, she persisted, in order to repair the deep hole left in her family with his infidelity. She worked to rebuild her self-esteem and get over the guilt she had at not being "good enough." It certainly helped that she met me. Now despite occasional forays into self-doubt due to situations like today, she seemed fine. Well-adjusted. Loving.

Maybe I *should* go with her. Once wouldn't kill me. Well, it might. But bottom line—she'd handed me a key to understand her better. What man in his right mind would turn that down?

She somehow got us in to see her psychologist that

same week.

***

The receptionist ushered us into the office. Sharon slipped into a tan upholstered seat. I heaved my huge frame into a second one beside her. I thrust my hand out. "Joe Belan." The psychologist took it in his firm grasp, and shook it. By the end of that first session, I had a grudging respect for the man.

As soon as we left the office, Sharon was all smiles, saying, "Didn't I tell you this one was different? Didn't I, now? I did!" She clapped her hands. "You *like* him, I can tell."

"I don't know if I'd go *that* far but yes, I'll give the counseling a shot."

"Whew! You'll see. It'll be worth it. It'll help us as a couple."

We learned how to overcome shadows—triggers from the past that color the present. I didn't even think we had a problem with that but lo and behold, we did. We both had a lot to overcome. We discovered some of the nuts and bolts of our weird psyches, and how to avoid bringing out the worst in ourselves. He taught us how to communicate, not only by listening but also by learning to read each other's body language. By the end of a year, I had made a 180 degree turnaround.

We still got on each other's nerves once in awhile, but the counselor gave us great tools to work with and provided the background we needed to succeed—as he said, "to press more good buttons than bad."

I vowed to send Sharon a different arrangement of flowers every month till school let out. *I'll give that Paul a little competition.* She was *my* favorite teacher in the world, too.

Sharon continued to improve. Aside from the long, mostly-silent drive to Magee in Pittsburgh once a month to be tested, our lives seemed calm. We'd breathe a sigh of relief when Dr. Clemente pronounced her "cancer-free" once again. The ride home passed more rapidly, with Sharon chattering away and demanding we stop to take photos of scenery as inspiration for her paintings.

We began to see longer stretches of green and shorter patches of white as March arrived. Gloves were left home as often as we took them. It could only get better from here on out. *Can't wait to get out on the golf course again.*

Sharon picked a piece of lint off a green pair of pants and held a banner in her hand that said *Kiss me, I'm Irish.* "Tomorrow is St. Paddy's Day," she said with a gleam in her eye. "You know what *that* means?"

"If you don't wear green, you get pinched?"

"Well, yes, but that's not what I'm referring to."

"I know….you're thinking of your mother's annual green drink."

"You got it. That wonderful rum slush drink she makes. By the way, she's having her party tomorrow night and we're invited."

"Oh my God, Sharon, that drink always makes me think of Cindy's loopy green teeth grin at the wedding reception we had at your mom's place. I'll never forget it."

Erie, 1999

We had found some Glenn Miller swing music dance medleys and had just finished dancing to *Little Brown Jug.* Out of breath, we flopped down on a sofa in the family room. Loud laughter drifted in through the open windows.

We looked at each other then pulled back the curtains to peer out onto the patio. That sounded like Cindy,

Burney's wife. Sharon's sister made her way inside and reported. "Cindy is experiencing Mom's famous green rum slush. She's had about five or six of those green bombs."

We took a walk outside. Cindy was dancing all by herself, staggering and smiling her big, beautiful smile, displaying bright green teeth, and gums. She blew a kiss with her equally green lips.

"That's our Cindy," I said.

Sharon giggled. "God bless her. She's celebrating for us."

St. Paddy's Day, which, for a city its size, a whole lot of people in Erie celebrate, finally arrived. Shar planned a day of "green" activities in her classroom. After work, we got in on the action with happy hour at Molly Brannigans, then went on to her mother's place to partake of the annual green drink. Her mother held court as she recounted the highlights of the parade downtown.

"I'm surprised someone doesn't dump green dye in Lake Erie," I observed. "The mayor of San Antonio dyes the river green every year. The city has a parade right there on the San Antonio River that winds through the Riverwalk. God, you can't even move. I'm surprised no one ever falls into the river with all the happy hours that take place in the little restaurants along the Riverwalk."

Paula, Sharon's sister, snorted. "That's funny. Don't they speak Spanish there? How many true-blue Irish live in San Antonio?"

Sharon's mum stuck a green tongue at me. "Ha. Lake Erie's already green from all the algae in the water."

"Grandma, it looks like you have some green algae on your tongue," joked Matt.

"Ahhh, the magic properties of that glorious green slushy rum drink." I laughed.

After a few rounds of *Danny Boy* and *Irish Eyes are*

Smilin,' we called it a night.

The days sped on to summer. We still had our once-a-month trip to Magee to contend with. We didn't look forward to it, considering the purpose in going. Would the test for the CA-125 levels in Sharon's blood remain negative (and Sharon cancer-free) or would it show up positive, pushing the levels up into danger again?

"Honey, your hair has grown out so much that you really don't need to wear a wig anymore. We need to celebrate that, don't we?"

"I just feel better today wearing it," she said fidgeting with papers in the glove box of the car.

"What are you looking for?"

She closed the dash. "Nothing, just nervous energy."

"Make sure the proof of insurance and the registration don't get lost," I intoned. "I'm rather obsessive about knowing where all the important documents are stored in the glove box in case I need to retrieve them. I like them to be in a particular order."

She glared at me and snapped the glove compartment closed.

I wanted to soften my words but nothing came to mind immediately.

Once we got to the hospital, Sharon went into the examination room and put on one of those ugly green hospital gowns.

I looked over at her. "Whoever named those monstrosities 'gowns' should be flogged."

She rolled her eyes and calmly said, "I guess they serve their purpose."

A nurse came by to collect her blood and carried the vials away for testing. Dr. Clemente awed us as he entered the room with a flourish. Specialists like him go out of their way to keep the hope alive for their patients.

He set his clipboard down and said exuberantly, "How's everybody doing this month?"

"Couldn't be better, doc." I had a big smile.

The doctor turned to Sharon, "Ready? Let's see how things are going." She lay down and he quickly and efficiently completed a physical and continued with an internal exam. As he finished up, he asked if we had any questions. As usual, Sharon had eight or nine lined up.

When Dr. Clemente left the room, she tossed the horrible gown on the table and put her clothes back on. He'd usually come bouncing in, all smiles and we'd know that Sharon continued to be cancer-free for another month. This time, the doctor came into the room looking somber and more serious than usual. Gone was his flashy smile and effusive movements.

Sharon and I stared at each other. Would today be different than each of the preceding ten visits? Had our luck run out?

"I'm afraid I have some bad news." Dr. Clemente explained that her numbers had risen to 280. "To give you an idea of the severity of this reading, let me tell you what her reading was last month—0.001."

A million thoughts ran through my mind. Were we going to be thrown into the same drama as before? Oh God. I looked around the room that suddenly seemed to shrink. I saw Sharon leaning against the examining table trying to control her emotions, and the doctor standing nearby as he held his clipboard with the damn numbers. The solemn expression remained on his face as he waited…for what? Us to react?

There's an expression, "Don't shoot the messenger." By God, that's exactly what I wanted to do as the doctor delivered the news. I knew logically that it wasn't his fault. But there had to be a culprit. I could feel my heart sink.

How many months of this could we stand? What was the prognosis? How many more rounds of chemo would we need? I thought back to Sharon's earlier nervousness? Did she have a sixth sense the news would be bad today?

Sharon let out a long sigh. "What's next?" I moved to her side ready to support her. Again, we would face this together.

I could hear the obligatory words doctors say to give patients hope. He told us about several treatments that had proven successful in clinical trials. I know this is part of his job but the words seemed hollow to me. We nodded through it all and got the scrip for Sharon's continued chemo treatments.

As we exited the office, I glimpsed the doctor as he rounded the corner. He suddenly seemed like any other man. He'd lost that greater-than-life aura. I remembered how Sharon even looked at his name as a good sign. Now I pictured him more like the Wizard of Oz hiding behind an illusionary curtain. The gifted surgeon in his element nearly always delivered the first time around. As long as the cancer stayed away, the curtain remained in place. But take away the curtain, you'd find a mere man at a control board.

'Pay no attention to that man behind the curtain. The great and powerful Wizard of Oz has spoken.'

Chapter 9
RIDING THE STORM

Upon our return home, our family, friends and several of Sharon's co-workers called to ask about the outcome of the tests. Ironically, they asked more now than in the past ten months combined, as if they already knew this time would be different.

We needed time to sort through our feelings, absorb the news and evaluate our options. The sympathy would come. The questions would follow. We didn't have any answers yet. A weekend home alone, just the two of us, gave us our broad game plan: fight the cancer. If anyone could beat it, Sharon could.

"OK, Shar, you got the ball here. You're the quarterback and the only one who can make the winning touchdown. Of course, teamwork is essential. It's only going to work if you hand off the ball to me when you get tired, and let me run with it until you get the energy to take it up again. Got it?" I thought for a minute. "We'll have a whole team helping you, honey. Rule #1: trust your gut and your teammates. We got your back."

"We can't lose if God is our coach," She said with fervor.

Call me selfish but deep in my heart I wanted her to fight because I couldn't bear the thought of losing her. I wanted her on my team—the winning team—for a long time yet. In order for that to happen, she had to make the last touchdown. My mind kept going back to our marriage vow, "to have and to hold." I wanted to live out those words.

A few days later, a double-whammy hit us. After my radical prostatectomy in 1999, I had to have my blood tested every three months. Now routine, I didn't think anything of it until I received a phone call from Dr.

Newton, my cancer specialist in Pittsburgh. It had been

nearly a year since I talked to him. Of course, he asked

about Sharon the first thing. As I explained to him what

we'd just learned, he groaned.

"Ah, that makes my job all the more difficult."

"Pardon?"

"Joe, I hate to tell you this, buddy, but your cancer

came back, too."

I clenched my teeth and shook my head back and forth,

as if doing so would erase the doctor's words. Every curse

word I knew came to mind, but I had the presence not to

vocalize them. I started to pace. "You mean to tell me that

not only does Sharon have to fight like hell, I've got to face

my own battle?"

"Sure looks like it, Joe. Damn cancer's got

everybody." After I stopped railing, I asked him how I

should proceed. "The best course of action would be for you to relocate in Pittsburgh during the week. Come to the hospital. We'll set you up with a series of radiation treatments. The sooner you can start, the better. I know you're living in Erie now. That makes everything a little more difficult. Is there someone you can stay with while you're receiving the treatments?"

"Not a problem." I could set up camp at Burney's place. He lived close enough to commute to the hospital and back. If I timed it right, I'd miss the worst traffic.

"Joe, you know my number if you need to get hold of me. Make whatever arrangements you need to get this squared away for next week. Let me know if I can help you in any other way. If not, I'll see you at nine on Monday morning."

"Your office?"

"Yes, we'll take some time to go through the

paperwork, then get started with the radiation."

"I'll be there." I said more curtly than I intended.

Sharon was asleep. I dreaded having to tell her. I imagined the shocked expression on her face and the tears that would come. Even worse, she'd have to cope with her chemo alone. I continued to pace as I planned out the easiest way to let her in on this development.

In spite of my elaborate plans to cushion the blow, it turned out she'd overheard part of the conversation between Dr. Newton and me. "Joe, did I hear something about your cancer returning or was that a dream?"

"You mean a nightmare?"

"So, I *did* hear you correctly." She took a long deep breath. "Honey, we'll get through this, too." She took me in her arms, and we comforted each other as best we could. Finally, she said, "God will give us the strength to make it through each day. His grace is sufficient. Remember He's your coach, too."

"Who will help you stand all the emergencies?" I blurted out.

"Honey, listen to me. God promises to be with us no matter where we are or what we go through, right? He'll never make us go through anything alone. He tells us that right in the Bible, so we have to trust Him on that." She spoke, a little timidly, as if she were trying to convince herself. "Besides, you are going to have to take care of you right now."

"I don't know why this came up right now with me. Of all the times…" I said, angry and a little shell-shocked.

"No matter how much we want to help each other, I guess we can't always do that. This is one of those situations." Sharon bit her lip. She looked at me.

Did she expect me to just fall in line with what she was saying? I guess I could intellectually. But my gut didn't feel right about leaving her.

I touched her arm. "Aren't you afraid?"

"Sure, I am. Chemo is scary stuff. We went through so much the first time. It's hard—especially losing my hair." She patted her head with both hands as if to reassure herself she still had hair, at least for now.

"Well—"

"Remember you even said we had a lot of people on our team." She playfully shook a finger at me.

"We do." *But nobody can fight for you like I can.*

"And Jesus Christ, our head coach, won't let us down. He knows the opposition. He knows it's a big game and He's given me a lot of responsibility. I'm a quarterback in His plan. He'll outline the right plays. If we listen, we'll get it right." She smacked one fist into her hand for emphasis.

I looked at her in amazement. She seemed strong and convicted. "Can you show me where that's written?"

"The part about the game plan or the other?"

Laughingly, she left and came back leafing through the pages of her Bible. "Here it is—Romans 8:38-39. Basically it says that nothing will faze us unless we let it. Not life or death or angels or demons. Not the present nor the future. Nothing can separate us from God's love."

I attended Catholic school up until the sixth grade. I don't know what I learned there, but it didn't come close to the kind of everyday faith Sharon practiced.

I asked God for strength to take us through each of our treatments and to give us a long life together. I added at the very end, *P.S. God, help me to grow.*

***

I started my radiation treatments roughly the same time Sharon started with her chemotherapy at home in the

Regional Cancer Center. We'd talk several times a day. I didn't have any pain at all with the radiation. Dr. Newton said I was an anomaly in that respect. When I told my wife that I tolerated the radiation so well, she exclaimed, "Yes! That's a blessing from God and an answer to our prayers."

She had the same types of problems with chemo that she had earlier, but since I couldn't be there, family members and friends filled in for me and helped her out whenever they could. Our married life took on the same qualities our former long-distance dating period had consisted of—constant calls back and forth and a prized weekend together at the end of the week.

"I've been a good boy with my treatment," I'd say. "I get to come home this weekend."

Not long into our forced separation, Sharon made a decision. "I know we ate breakfast at *Taki's* and already celebrated our anniversary this past June but being separated all week, I'd like to plan something new and different. I thought it would be cool if we had a "Joe and Sharon wedding extravaganza," night while the weather is still nice. What do you think?"

I smoothed my moustache. "What exactly do have in mind?"

As she drew me onto the couch, I caught her enthusiasm. We'd invite an assortment of people to the house to celebrate with us. Our wedding extravaganza would begin on Friday at four. After a light dinner, everyone would sit down and view our wedding video. On Saturday, we'd have nachos and cheese, tacos and frozen margaritas in a Mexican-themed get together that would last a couple of hours to commemorate our Cancun honeymoon. The wheels kept turning as she outlined ideas. The sparkle in her eyes returned. *God, I loved her.*

She threw her arms around my neck. "I'm tired to

death of feeling sick. This'll give us something to look forward to. We'll dress up on Friday night. It'll be such fun."

I took her literally and frowned. "Where can I find a tuxedo at this time of year?"

"Tux-shmux. 'Smart casual' will work well for both of us. We just need a party mood to perk up our lives, and get rid of the yukky-feel from our treatments. How about next weekend? That'll give us time before we settle into the Steelers' season this fall, don't you think, Joe?"

It didn't matter what I thought. To see my wife's green eyes shine once again, I'd do pretty much anything she asked of me. "Let's just keep it as simple as we can." That chemo really took it out of her. "I think Friday night is enough. Remember we just don't know how you'll feel. Tell you what, if you do feel well enough, we'll just get in the car and drive on I-90 and find someplace to go. It'll be a quickie honeymoon," I said, ending with a persuasive kiss.

"Maybe you're right."

All week, we sneaked in urgent calls regarding food, guests, or the odd decoration. Our calls took on a whispered intimacy and I couldn't wait for the weekend to arrive. Those at the hospital where I got my radiation all knew about the extravaganza. Let's just say I got teased a lot. Friday morning, I squeezed in part of a treatment and planned to arrive back in Erie by noon.

Dr. Newton came in to shake my hand, "I hear that congratulations are in order, young man. Have an extravagant weekend and don't get too married," he admonished with a smile.

"You mean, *old* man, don't you?" I smoothed out my gray sideburns and moustache. *Man, sixty-four years old.* Not that I felt it, except after a day out on the golf course.

Sharon met me at the door, wearing a long black wig, a tank top, bell bottom blue jeans and sandals. She'd painted her toenails pink—radical for her. My mouth dropped open. "Have we gone back to the seventies, Shar?" Then it hit me, "I get it. Cher Bono." She tossed her sleek hair over one shoulder and began to sing an off-tune rendition of *I Got You, Babe*.

"Wait till I tell you our plans for this song tonight." As she bent over to whisper in my ear, all I could think of was how beautiful she looked in spite of her swollen face and chemo-ravaged body.

The weather cooperated fully with our plans. Guests came to celebrate the light-hearted "anniversary." Someone from church had made a banner. It now hung from a post at each end of the porch and riffled in the breeze. In big black letters it read, JOE & SHARON'S WEDDING EXTRAVAGANZA - 5 YEARS.

We offered salads, cold-cuts, snacks and drinks of all kinds. For a fee, one could even "buy" the famous green bomb wedding drink. We had twenty-three people in the house celebrating with us. "We're ready to dim the lights and pop in the video," Sharon's sister, Paula, shouted.

That was our cue. We entered the room in our Sonny and Cher ensemble. As we looked into each other's eyes, we sang our signature song *I Got You, Babe*. Our guests screamed in laughter. Shar was right. It set the perfect tone for the evening.

When we did pop the video in, with Sharon close to me, the dark room faded. Our wedding unfolded just as it did that summer day five years ago.

Erie, 1999

June 26, 1999, turned out to be an ideal wedding day, with temperatures in the mid 70s. We married at the Summit United Methodist Church where Sharon attended, with the Reverend Lou Palmer officiating. The small picturesque church suited us perfectly. We loved the cozy feel, the stain-glassed windows, the big steeple and its enormous Christmas fir in front. It also had ample parking for our guests.

For our ceremony, we had the forty or more guests stand in a semi-circle around the altar. We set it up so that there'd be someone from my side of the family next to someone from Sharon's side. Of course, we made sure there were seats for anyone unable to stand. Toward the end of the service, we joined hands in a beautiful communal prayer. We never felt so blessed.

Sharon and I wrote our own vows, which emphasized our love for Jesus and each other. I held both of her hands during the rites. She looked so radiant and happy that I wished I could have taken her in my arms instead of merely holding her hands. She said her vows flawlessly, but I stumbled and stuttered through mine. Both the Reverend and Sharon had to prompt me. My hands and knees quivered. Sharon looked at ease.

After we finished saying what we had in our hearts, Reverend Palmer took over with the traditional vows. I'd told Sharon earlier, "To have, to hold, in sickness and health, we're going to do all that stuff without being reminded or needing to say them in front of witnesses."

"Well, it won't hurt us to say 'em anyway. I want to hear these promises, too."

"Awww, I'll do it for you, Shar."

Now I was glad we'd made it part of our ceremony. We were holding hands, giddily gazing into each other's eyes when the Reverend threw in a curve ball. "Do you promise to give Sharon all of your retirement money, all of your social security checks, your Steelers tickets, and your golf clubs?"

"I *will*." I declared fervently, without realizing what I'd agreed to.

All our guests and even the Reverend burst out laughing, including me. I repeated, "I will."

Our close friend, Laura, played a mixture of wedding music and traditional Koinonia hymns on the organ. After the ceremony, we strolled back down the aisle in our first moments as husband and wife to the music of *I Got You Babe,* by Sonny and Cher. We went back to the altar to take some photos and give our guests time to load up on miniature bottles of bubbles to wish us well as we ran from the church.

Blue skies, green grass and clean air made for great bubble-making shots. Along with comfortable temperatures, we had a mild zephyr to toss and carry the bubbles in swirls around us. As well-wishers shook the bottles and showered us with tiny bubbles, I glowed with happiness for our future. Although I'd been married twice before, I never had such a certainty of how "right" Sharon was for me. And judging from her expression, she felt the same way. As I watched her through an aura of bubbles, she laughed and smiled. She must have been a bubble magnet because they would gravitate and kamikaze into her while giving me the once-around. Sunshine highlighted those beautiful bubble-filled moments. *Oh Shar, it's not just the sun in the sky, it's a heavenly light radiating from you, my sunshine.*

The video panned to the parking lot of the restaurant where we held our reception. Sharon and I got out of my car with a sign flapping on the back that said, "Wedded Bliss." The Station Break restaurant had a real dining car that stood on the railroad tracks. We'd arranged to have them serve steak, their signature dish, along with baked potatoes, a salad and vegetable. The eight-ounce marinated rib-eye was served to perfection. The toasts came in.

My best friend leveled a look in my direction. "What took you so long, Belan? Did the wear and tear of five years of driving finally convince you to put an end to that long-distance love?"

"This is not the end. Rather, it's the beginning," someone shouted.

"Amen to that," and a chorus of "Amens" followed.

Burney jabbed the microphone in my direction. "I'm bummed out you're moving once-and-for-all to Erie, but I can see you got a helluva great roommate."

"Sharon begged me to make an honest woman of her…"

She gave me a little shove. "Joe…"

As I caught her hand and brought it to my lips, our guests cheered. Cousin Dave shouted, "Uh-oh! Watch it, bud. Stick to the truth at least on your wedding day."

We held our reception at my mother-law's place in Wesleyville. Fortunately, we had clear skies, so the party continued outside on Ann's patio, spilling into the backyard. Our guests mingled together as if they'd known each other all their lives.

As the wedding video ended with Sharon and me dancing to that beautiful, bold swing music of Glenn Miller, I was reminded of our first dance together at the Gettysburg Social. I whispered, "You make a helluva dance partner, babe."

Just before her lips found mine, she whispered back, "You make a great roommate."

The next morning, we slept in to give Sharon more energy. The chemo just took it right out of her. I was relieved she went for my idea of a "fake" follow-up honeymoon instead of a party at the house. We loaded up the Explorer and headed for I-90.

Looking at each other, we shouted our launching cheer, "We're off on another Sharon-and-Joe's excellent adventure!" It might sound silly to other people, but it meant something to us. We'd say this whether we took off on a day trip or a longer vacation. It gave us the right mindset. We also had a ritual of listening to CDs along the way. We'd always put in *Shine, Jesus Shine.* Shar once said it made her feel that God was right there in the front seat with us on the journey. After she said that, it took on a special meaning and I'd put it in first. We also played a lot of Billy Joel, Buddy Holly, 1950s oldies and some bluegrass music.

We decided to keep driving until curiosity stimulated us to see something we'd never seen before. Billboard after billboard advertised *Bonner's Christmas Store* in Frankenmuth, Michigan. When we consulted the map, we came across some towns that sounded quaint, like

Marquette and Sault Ste. Marie, which would make it worth visiting Michigan's Upper Peninsula.

On our drive north, Sharon's ever-vigilant eyes spotted something she wanted to photograph, which might later make its way onto her paint canvas. "Stop, wait, wait, wait, turn around. I want to get a picture of those trees." She always pointed with her eyes, chin, and nose, and a nod of her head.

I spotted a break in the highway with a turn-around lane. As I sped up, we both saw a sign that said, "No U-turns." Sharon peered through the window. "Maybe we should continue on until we find a place where we can turn around."

I took a quick look, put on my turning signal and made the illegal U-turn. We drove on about a mile until we reached the trees my wife wanted to photograph. I was driving southbound in the slow lane. "Pull over on the berm, Joe."

She turned, looking over her shoulder to seek out the perfect place to stop and snap her photos. When we pulled over, I switched on my four-way flashers to warn other southbound travelers of our presence. Ironically, we'd halted right next to a sign that said, "No Stopping. Emergency vehicles only. Violators will be prosecuted."

Sharon walked toward the clump of trees shooting about forty or fifty photos. We didn't see any state boys, luckily, especially since we were about to the break the law for the third time in an hour by making another illegal U-turn to return to the northbound lane.

The things I do for this woman!

On Sunday morning we made our way to Mackinac Island. "From what it says on this brochure, they don't allow vehicles of any kind there," I observed. "Plus, I sure would like to see the Grand Hotel. It's featured in the movie, *Somewhere In Time*, you know that love story with Christopher Reeve and Jane Seymour." Their story kind of reminded me of my love for Sharon.

When we made it to the Grand Hotel, I took in the grandeur of the world's largest front porch. "Shar, this historic hotel opened all the way back in 1887. Can you believe it? It's everything I imagined. Look at the lake. Do you want to sit on the rocking chair for a few minutes to enjoy the view?"

She nodded, as awestruck as I was. Our tour of the hotel ended with a lunch buffet. I couldn't say enough great things about it. In my opinion, the Grand Hotel was the highlight of the island visit.

Much better than some of the other aspects of the island, like the crush and jostling of people elbowing their way from shop to shop. Since horses served as the main mode of transportation on the island, horse manure covered the streets, so we had to carefully navigate around. The smell began to permeate our clothing so that even when we temporarily escaped the manure, we could still smell it. The worst, nasty black flies constantly swarmed around our faces, causing us to swat and slap at ourselves the whole time. The bold flies stuck to us. Sometimes we even had to snap at them to get them to fly away.

As we left the island, we bought some fudge, our only souvenir. Back in the car, I took it out of the bag and casually read the label. "Ha! Shar, guess what? Our genuine Mackinac fudge really comes from the kitchens of Erie, PA." *Go figure.*

It took us twelve hours to drive home. We arrived early Monday morning, completely exhausted. "Honey, we're both going to have to play hooky from our treatments today. We're in no shape to do anything. Besides, I can't drive another mile."

For a minute, Sharon looked guilty like a schoolgirl about to skip a class in which she had a test scheduled. Would the principal catch her doing this dastardly deed? The torn look on her face almost made me change my mind, except my aching body screamed, *That's enough!*

As we curled up together in bed, I said, "Happy fake honeymoon."

"Fake? Seemed real to me. At least we got *genuine* Mackinac fudge out of the deal."

Immediately after Sharon learned her cancer had come back, we started researching online for oncologists, hospitals and the American Cancer Society. We felt we'd gone as far as we could go with Magee and wanted new hope. One day she returned from school with a big smile and some information. "Joe, I was talking to my friend, Lisa. She has a sister who works at the Children's Hospital in Houston who speaks glowingly about the wonderful, miraculous work being done at M.D. Anderson Cancer Hospital. She even gave us a phone number."

We stared at each other and simultaneously said, "The Lord works in mysterious ways."

Sharon jumped on her computer and googled it. If we could believe the hype of their ads, the state-of-the-art procedures they performed led to a phenomenal amount of successes and cancers cured. Highly regarded, the doctors came from all over the world as did the staff and patients. Still, M D Anderson didn't make our first cut. We narrowed down our top two choices to Roswell Park Cancer Institute in Buffalo and the Cleveland Clinic. At that point, we only considered hospitals within a three-hundred-mile radius of Erie.

But things changed rapidly when Sharon discovered more advantages of M.D. Anderson. She had a thing about positive "signs." She believed that whenever we face many choices, God tips the scales by sending a sign to let us know that's the one we should choose. It was her way—and now mine—of confirming that we made the right choice.

First of all, she found out that M.D. Anderson was a straight shot, route-wise, to where her son, Matt, lived and taught. What's more, her sister's family lived right in Houston, not far from the hospital.

We thought more about this last option over the next few days and decided to follow up with a phone call. It seemed another good sign when we actually received a live person on the other end of the switchboard who transferred us to the *head office* of the top ovarian specialist there. We couldn't believe it. Although the oncologist, Dr. Judith Lobo, couldn't talk to us right then, the administrative assistant promised she'd return our call at five o'clock that afternoon. A call-back! We'd never had one of those before.

We discussed the matter that afternoon over coffee. I

set my cup down, taking a napkin to wipe up some that sloshed over the top, and I turned to Sharon "What do you think about this whole thing in Houston?"

"I don't know. I'm getting excited. I somehow feel that we need to pursue this lead. It's giving me good vibes. They seem so knowledgeable and professional, and very helpful."

"Wouldn't you rather be somewhere closer to home?"

She shrugged. "Maybe that shouldn't be our biggest consideration. Feeling comfortable with the hospital and the practitioners who work with your case is more important. I guess it all depends on if she actually calls us back or not, and how she comes across on the phone."

"What if we like her, and she gives the green light, should we go for it?"

"I think God was speaking through my friend." She picked up a chocolate chip cookie to dunk in her coffee.

"Yes, by all means, if God opens the door, we have to walk through it."

"If you're convinced, I am, too."

At precisely five o'clock, the phone rang. We looked at each other. Sharon laughed. "*Another* good sign."

After Dr. Lobo introduced herself, I picked up the extension and we had a detailed three-way conversation about Sharon's condition. Dr Lobo either had an eidetic memory or tape recorded the conversation because she never slowed down or paused to take notes. She came across as caring and professional. Even so, Sharon saved her key and most frequently-asked question for last. "Have you ever known anyone with recurrent ovarian cancer to beat it?"

"Oh, sure." She said. "We do it all the time."

Sharon caught her breath and asked boldly. "When can I come then?" Up until this point, all our doctors had said *no one* had beaten it. Given our situation, she had one, maybe two years left.

"Let's get you scheduled for preliminary tests."

Our eyes met and I nodded. *Go for it.* "Make that touchdown, babe," I whispered.

Her green eyes sparkled as she gave me two thumbs up.

Dr. Lobo would transfer the records from Magee Women's Hospital. That left us to gather all the paperwork regarding Sharon's treatment from the Regional Cancer Center in Erie.

My wife handled everything that had to do with the paperwork and arranged for a two-week leave of absence from school. She kept everyone involved in the loop. I took care of the travel logistics, including maps, a check-up by our mechanic, Trip-Tiks from AAA, preparing the vehicle and packing the car.

One and a half weeks later on September 25th, 2004, we slid into the car. As we backed out, we checked to ensure that the garage door closed securely.

"Sharon, see that garage door go down? That's reminds me of our life right now."

"What do you mean?"

"After thirty-eight doses of radiation, my cancer's in remission. I'm sure you'll get positive results, too. I believe our past challenges will disappear behind that door and future success awaits us in Houston."

"So it's like a curtain closing at the end of a scene on a play."

"Yes, exactly! You got it. We just have to wait to see what this scene brings us."

Toward the end of our drive, I discovered something about my wife that surprised the heck out of me. I never knew she had such an overactive imagination or that she could be so obstinate. This little side adventure highlighted the differences in our personalities more than any other journey we'd taken together.

We were driving along US State Route 59 in Texas when we came across what appeared to be an automobile junkyard. The sign scrawled in runny, black paint read, "Open for Business, Only." What was that supposed to mean? Sharon wanted to take a photograph of the sign but couldn't get it from the right angle so we had to turn around and go back.

Even though we slowed down as we came around the bend, we still missed the proper angle. I didn't want to back up on the hilly, curvy road so I decided to travel further south, find a turnaround and come up on the junkyard from the other side. That way we could get out of the car, walk around and take as many shots as we wanted. Still morning, the sun was perfectly positioned at our backs.

When I stopped the car on the berm of the highway, Sharon hissed at me, "Keep going, keep going, keep going." Alarmed by her tone and some unknown danger Sharon must have seen, I checked the rear and side-view mirrors for potential hazards and floored the gas pedal. The tires threw up bits of sand and stones as I sped away.

"What…what…what? What's the matter?" I hissed back.

She smacked my arm. "Did you see those two stretch limos sitting in the driveway?"

"Yes, er, no, I mean, so what? Why are we whispering?"

"Don't you think there was something wrong with that picture?"

I gripped the steering wheel in irritation. "No, why don't you tell me."

Sharon gave me a litany of danger she found in that scene. With her fingers, she ticked off each point, still whispering. "An eight-foot cyclone fence lined with sheets of corrugated steel blocking the view, and topped with razor wire guarding the place. Somebody wants to keep prying eyes out and the *owners* of those prying eyes from getting in. They probably have dogs and security cameras."

"Shar, come on—" She placed her hand in front of my mouth to shush me.

I found a place to turn around even though she continued arguing. "What about the two big black shiny out-of-place limousines with black tinted windows parked inside the fence? Hmm? And that sign...it's too subtle. Why didn't they put "Trespassers Keep Out" with skull and crossbones for extra measure? It's also out in the middle of nowhere. So you see..."

I started to recognize the landmarks as we came to the

junkyard again. "Bullcrap. Let's take the picture anyway."
Fearlessly, I pulled across the driveway entrance and
ordered, "Take the picture."

She refused and turned her back away from the limos.
With her arms folded defiantly, she tucked the camera
under her breast. No way was I going to wrestle the camera
from her. We sat there, defying each other with our
'Mexican Stand-off' postures until I relented and drove
away, returning to US Route 59 South toward Houston.

We both let out big sighs, mine of resignation, hers of
relief as we continued south to meet our destiny.

Finally, she said, "I had a baaad feeling about that
place. You are always reckless."

"Oh come on."

"Yes, you are. Just like a teenager."

"I've got to hand it to you there but for completely
different reasons than what you're thinking. I've always got

raging hormones." I caressed her leg and gave her a sidelong glance meant as a peace offering.

She allowed for a fleeting smile to land on her lips before she turned serious again. For the next fifty miles, I caught her checking the mirrors for pursuing limos. That one hour delay in our driving time gave us many hours of debate, discussion and nervous speculation. To this day, I wish that Sharon had taken that picture.

Once we arrived at M.D. Anderson Cancer Center, we registered. There, we received a packet of information intended to help patients navigate through the labyrinth of halls and specialized departments. I have a dead-reckoning sense of direction, but we got lost several times. It didn't take long to register that more than fifty thousand people worked in this huge facility that ranked as one of the top cancer centers in the United States, if not *the* best, in the world.

At the Ovarian Cancer Oncology Department, the receptionist ushered us into the conference room to meet Dr. Judith Lobo and another oncologist, Dr. Lorraine Rose. We hand delivered the x-rays and radiological prints taken in Pittsburgh and Erie. The two doctors had already received the pathology slides from Pittsburgh confirming the cancer in Sharon's tissues that the Pittsburgh pathologists could not find.

As they bombarded us with information, we scribbled furiously so that later we could sort through it and ask intelligent questions. As it turned out, we didn't need to do that because the hospital had yet another pamphlet that included all that kind of information. Our heads spun at how fast all this was happening—all God's providence, according to my wife. "There is no doubt in my mind that God supplied all the right people and technology in the best place at the right time," Sharon whispered, awed.

After several days of testing, the doctors met with us again. We learned that Sharon was an excellent candidate for a clinical trial they had for stem cell transplant *if* they could get her cancer into a complete remission and if she could pass some more tests. We had ten months to get Sharon cancer-free to participate. We'd accomplish that at the Regional Cancer Center in Erie.

We left M.D. Anderson convinced that getting this stem cell procedure was the right thing to do, not only because God led us here but also because of our faith that He would make a miracle. After all, one of our mottos was, "We believe in miracles."

Sharon pulled out her Bible as we got going on the road. "Listen, honey," Sharon said, a peaceful look in her eyes. "Mark 11:22-24 promises, 'If anyone says to this mountain, go throw yourself into the sea, and does not doubt in his heart but believes that what he says will happen, it will be done for him. Therefore, I tell you whatever you ask in prayer, believe that you receive it and it will be yours.'"

"That's right."

She continued. "So, I pray for healing and claim that verse."

Her faith continually amazed me. As a result, her perspective began to rub off on me.

After more tests and several months of chemo that put Sharon in remission, we phoned Dr. Lobo to see if she were now eligible to participate in the clinical trial. *All systems go!*

God slipped the last detail in place when our insurance company stepped in to cover the procedure. We'd been prepared to mortgage the house but we didn't have to worry about that anymore.

I took Sharon's arm and twirled her around. Giddy

with excitement, we danced to whatever song I had in my head. As I held my wife of nearly seven years, I never felt more love for her than at that moment. We would beat this thing. She would make her touchdown.

Chapter 10
JOURNEYS

We still had a few months to wait before M.D. Anderson ran the stem cell trial. The cold affected Sharon, so I arranged for us to travel to New Smyrna Beach, Florida, and stay in a condominium in February and March 2005. This way, we'd escape the bad weather and dismal overcast skies of northwest Pennsylvania.

Sharon had gotten final clearance on disability leave for the second year in a row. After the chemo, she never fully recovered her rapid memory recall or all her strength. The memory lapses frustrated her in both preparing her lessons and teaching them, while not being able to lift anything hindered her classroom management. She missed her students, but this freed her up to travel.

I wanted to fly down to Florida but Sharon wouldn't

hear of it. "No, I want to see this country of ours, not just get there. It's all part of our adventure. I want to look at the scenery and take photos. It's not all about the destination. It's all about the experience of getting there."

"We can do all that in Florida and have sunshine, too," I protested.

Shar crossed her arms and stared me down. I couldn't hold out long when she used that tactic. "All right, all right. We'll drive."

"You're not going to change your mind?"

"No, I give you my word. Cross my heart and hope to
—"

With a fierce look, she interrupted, "Don't you dare say *die*."

Oh my God. The air went out of me as I turned away. I held my temples in horror. *What was I thinking?* We centered all our thoughts on *living*.

I turned back. "I'm so sorry, honey. I didn't mean that at all."

"I know you didn't." She whispered. "I just don't want to tempt fate."

***

We traveled uneventfully from Erie through all of the states from Pennsylvania to 'West, by God,' Virginia into Virginia. As crossed over the Carolinas, Sharon shouted, "Hcy, slow down, or stop for a minute! I need to take a photo of this 'LEAVING NORTH CAROLINA' sign." Five minutes later, she said, "Wait! Hold on. Here it is! 'WELCOME TO SOUTH CAROLINA.'" She did this the whole way to Florida. I got a kick out it and made a game out of who could spot the state sign first.

I wanted to do the typical male thing, drive as fast as

the law allowed and not stop until we reached our final destination, in this case, Florida. I only wanted to break for gas and necessities. I got my driving motto from Admiral Farragut, an American war hero who proclaimed, "Damn the torpedoes. Full speed ahead." This must have frustrated the bejesus out of Sharon but she'd only frown when she felt that a point needed to be made.

She liked everything that had to do with nature and wanted to stop and admire it, especially rocks and rock formations, twisted, gnarly trees, and old barns and houses set off in the distance. For a keen observer like my wife, these "photo-ops" served as a smorgasbord of scenery for her artistic palette. On the other hand, I liked when the rubber met the road and made that whump-whump sound when it passed over the expansion joints in the road, and the spinning odometer as it tracked the distance traveled.

"Look at that!" she'd shout. I'd shift my gaze from the

road to wherever she was pointing and try to get a fix on it. By the time I figured it out at seventy miles per hour, the moment for sharing had passed. Our frustrations grew after each missed moment.

"Shar, we're like two amoebas that absorb each other's cultures," I observed our second day into the journey. "I'm scientific and you're artistic."

"Hmmm, good point." Her voice turned silky sweet and she spoke persuasively. "Try to *move* more like an amoeba. Have you ever seen a fast amoeba? 'Course not. *Slooow* down so you can absorb everything we're seeing. It's not a race. You're missing the best parts of the trip."

Maybe she was right. I agreed to take it easy on the gas pedal and stop for her frequent photo-ops. After she finished, I'd put the car into fast forward and aim for our Florida target again. As I concentrated on the road, she kept up a running commentary on the scenery.

"Joe, let's make a calendar of all the cool things we come across," she said, all excited. "We'll choose the twelve best photos. People will love them."

"That's a great idea."

She spotted several clouds, especially ones with sun rays peeking through. At one point, we saw a hundred-foot high cross. Sharon also came across some road signs like one that read, 'USED COWS FOR SALE.' We tried to imagine what a used cow looked like. On US Route 59, we saw a sign in front of a run-down house surrounded by detritus that read, 'JUNK FOR SALE, CHEEP.' We laughed at their spelling of cheap.

A huge old, gnarly oak tree growing in the middle of an endless pasture particularly fascinated Shar. She said, "It looks like an ancient, beaten warrior still standing tall and protecting its field from invaders." Maybe she saw me as a personification of the tree standing there giving her shade and protection. I like to think so anyway.

I tried to give her time to take her photographs. The more I played the patient husband, the more I started to genuinely enjoyed the journey.

Sharon and I seemed more in tune with each other somehow. Could it be that I was actually becoming less obsessed about getting somewhere as soon as I could in order to "relax"? Could I actually be learning to relax along the way? Was Sharon's perspective rubbing off on me? I've always been concerned with taking the most expedient route in getting anything done. That goes against the grain of being a science teacher. But maybe I was changing or at least heading in the right direction.

As Shar pointed yet again, "Look at the way the sun is shining through those weeds near that swamp. Oh honey, stop. If I can just capture…"

I smiled to myself as I pulled off the road. "You got it,

babe." *Imagine that, I am actually finding beauty in swamps instead of focusing on my scientific curiosity about alligators and snakes.*

The beachfront condo we stayed at in Florida belonged to Burney's brother who offered it to us for as long as we wanted to stay.

"Look Joe, the sky is so clear." Shar jumped out of the car and I followed.

She held out her arms and lifted her face to take in the sunshine, seeming to drink it in. "It must be in the mid-seventies. Ohhhh. My first time seeing the Atlantic Ocean. Feel the sea, I mean, *ocean* breeze coming off the water. Aaah. Smell the air. It's salty and there's some other distinct smell I can't quite place. But just perfect." She wrinkled her nose to try to distinguish what it could be.

That made me laugh. "Honey, you looked like a rabbit

just now."

"A rabbit, huh?" She twitched her nose, wiggled her index fingers, which magically became rabbit ears and smoothed imaginary whiskers. Then her smile gave way and she looked, just ... content.

Seeing the ocean through her eyes made me wish I could serve everything to her on a platter—the sun, water, waves, sand, walks, talks... I couldn't *wait* to begin our time together. How we *needed* this time to let loose and let wonder take over. "By the way, that peculiar odor is due to the marine life in the ocean."

"I like the smell of the Atlantic Ocean. It's ... fresh."

"I'd like go 'get' fresh," I raised an eyebrow suggestively.

Out by the car we stretched. *We had all the time in the*

world. I officially welcomed her to the Atlantic Ocean with a kiss. "Let's leave our luggage in the truck for now. We can come back and get it later."

"Joe, listen to the sounds of the surf and sea gulls calling to each other." From the parking garage under the condo, we listened and savored the moment. Afterward, we made our way up to Jerry's condo on the fifteenth floor.

I unlocked the door. "Come on, sweetheart." I took her hand and we made our way through the condo to the balcony. "This terrace overlooks the beautiful blue Atlantic Ocean," I said as if I were her personal tour guide. With the sun directly over our heads, I stood behind her, arms holding her as my body pressed hers to the railing. To our left in the hazy distance, we saw Daytona. Directly below our balcony and slightly to the left of the condo lay a park with a nature boardwalk snaking through it. I rubbed my thumb and forefinger together and said, "Even the air is different by the ocean. Can you feel it? It's moister."

"Yes, I can. Oh. Look at the pelicans. They look so graceful. How can they fly so close to the water but not fall in? They're landing. Look at them try to dodge the breaking surf. I'd like to see them catch a fish." She looked off in the distance and shaded her eyes. "*This* is living."

We thought the idyllic weather would continue for the whole two months.

Boy, did we get that wrong. The combination of storms in the Atlantic, and an Alberta Clipper pushing down from Canada caused the temperatures to plummet into the thirties and forties with rain and bone-chilling wind the very next day.

We languished in Jerry's luxurious living room for three weeks. We gazed out at the gray ocean under the gray overcast sky, which obliterated any chance of seeing a sunset or a sunrise.

I shook my head in frustration. "Every day is the same. This is not the Florida I wanted to show you." *How come the weather has to be so crappy?* She'd suffered so much already. We intended this trip to serve as an introduction to all the good things that would happen as a result of the stem cell procedure. I imagined it as the sunlight leading to an ever-warming future to fulfill that to-have-and-to-hold clause in our wedding vows. Instead, the raw weather outdoors prevented the leisurely romantic walks I envisioned us taking on the raised boardwalk that wound its way through the tropical beach flora.

"We did have that gorgeous first day," Sharon pointed out. "I had the perfect introduction to the Atlantic Ocean. I'm not at all disappointed. What if I'd never seen it at all?"

We took a break from the ugly weather by attempting a day trip to Miami. We got about halfway there before we decided to turn around and return to New Smyrna, taking in some of the local craft markets and restaurants.

We also took a trip to a place called the Holy Land Experience, not to be confused with "the holy land." There, we saw professionals re-enact stories from the Bible. We couldn't believe how realistic their performances were. Other side trips included touring an alligator reserve and taking an air boat ride through the Everglades. Of course, we couldn't miss Disneyworld or the Arabian Nights, which we saw for the first time.

"Sweetheart, the weather is nothing like what I hoped it would be for you here. Let's go west to Orlando."

Sharon agreed. Five weeks of cold weather had taken their toll on her. "Sounds like a good time to meet up with friends. We're lucky to have so many Erie friends to visit."

We locked up the condo and headed out. We talked a lot about the upcoming stem cell procedure on the leisurely drive to Houston. We had a pretty good idea of what Sharon would face, and it was daunting, to say the least. But we tried to bolster our confidence any time we talked about it.

"Sharon, you have the courage of a lion. You have whatever it takes to save your life. You have it. Remember you are the quarterback, and we are all part of your team."

She bit her bottom lip. "I'm not really that brave or skillful, honey, but with you beside me and God's protection, I can do it. I can make it."

"If I could, I'd go through the procedure for you." I let out a deep sigh.

She reached over and took my hand. "I know you would, Joe."

I thought if I could distract her, she wouldn't be so nervous. "Honey, do you want to stop and take a walk? Look at the ocean."

"No, I'm fine. Maybe I should. I probably won't be able to leave my room the whole time I'm in Houston, will I? What do you think about…"

Maybe if she can get this nervous chatter out, she'll be able to relax. Maybe she has to come to grips with the entire procedure.

"Honey, can we pull over and pray for me?" she asked.

"Of course we can." I said. As we pulled over, I put on my four-ways and holding hands we prayed for the success of the procedure. Sharon finished up. "…God let me be ready for whatever I need to face. Help me to understand everything and be courageous. In Jesus' name, Amen."

We swung across the Florida panhandle heading westward toward Gulfport, Mississippi, and the hurricane-ravaged coast. We were on our way to visit my friend Don Roberts and his wife, Janice. We wanted to observe firsthand what "Katrina" had done. We'd seen lots of footage on television, but the impact of seeing trees and homes uprooted by the backwash of the gulf made us appreciate the courage of the people who'd survived. The waters along with the debris receded into the shallower tide and floated off shore, as though mocking the residents of Gulfport and Biloxi who struggled to put their lives and homes back together.

We felt their pain. In a way, it symbolized what Sharon and I were going through. The ovarian cancer had ripped through Sharon's ovaries like Katrina and dared us to try to repair the damage. Several times along the way we had to pull to the side of the road to get a grip on the tears that suddenly started flowing. Each time we prayed for the people who'd had their homes ripped away by Katrina.

As we left the ravaged areas behind, we somberly headed into the biggest challenge of our lives. I wondered just how many more trips we'd have time to share together. Would she beat the odds? Or would the cancer return and silently steal her away from me? No doubt the devastated landscape contributed to my darker, more pessimistic thoughts. I looked over at my normally bubbly wife. She'd closed her eyes and sat uncharacteristically still. I slipped my hand over hers and squeezed it. "You okay?"

She seemed to be harnessing strength. When she looked at me, she said, "God is in the process of rebuilding their lives, and ours, too. We know, firsthand, that our world can change overnight. Ordinary things we take for granted can be lost. When we look at the damage, it seems overwhelming." She opened up her arms in response to all we'd just seen in New Orleans. "We need to focus on Him, and not our circumstances. He is *Jehova Jireh*, Our Great

Provider. Let's not lose our focus, Joe."

It was as if she'd read my mind earlier and God was speaking through her to me. I tried to swallow a big lump in my throat. Thank God an exit ramp appeared because I needed to pull off the busy highway to collect myself. "I'm here for you, babe. I'm focused again."

We pulled into an Exxon station and decided to take a short break. While I filled the tank, Shar walked into the store to buy some snacks for the road. As she walked away, I looked up and said, "God, if You loved me enough to send me Sharon, I'll trust You enough not to take her away."

Chapter 11
TOUGH CHALLENGES

Sharon and I got into Houston late in the morning and stopped off to see her sister. We chatted about Katrina and how long it would take to rebuild New Orleans. Conversation moved on to the stress of day-to-day living.

As usual, Shar shifted the topic to the positive. "Darlene, I can't believe I got into the hospital here. I know it's where God wants me to be."

"M.D. Anderson is renowned for its mission to rid the world of cancer," I added, just in case anyone had missed hearing me say it any of the ten times since they selected Sharon to be part of this clinical study.

Jon, Darlene's husband, lathered his hands under a steady stream of water at the kitchen sink. He spoke over the noise. "Can someone fill me in here? What kind of study is this?"

I jumped in. "It's called *stem cell gene therapy*. We've heard many good things about the results so far."

"Jon, get a towel," she said, flipping a burger on the stove. "You're dripping on my kitchen floor." She turned back to us. "How does that procedure work again?"

Sharon jerked a finger in my direction. "Ask him. Joe explains it best."

I eased into my science teacher mode. "Stem cell replacement therapy is pretty straightforward. Doctors harvest stem cells made in our bone marrow to fight any foreign invaders ranging from splinters to flu germs to cancer cells. Stem cells are really baby blood cells that enter the body's blood and lymphatic systems and become whatever component of blood the body needs. If they become white blood cells, they attack any abnormal cell or organism that infects the host body. The procedure is to harvest as many stem cells as possible from the host who donates them. When a person donates his own stem cells for their procedure, it's called *autologous*." I was itching to illustrate my explanation on an erasable board. Old habits die hard.

"And that's what Sharon's getting, right? Autogolous. So that means, um, that she's donating her own stem cells … to herself?"

"That's right."

"Brave girl." Her sister set the spoon down and gave Sharon a hug. "We know you'll give it all you have, no pun intended"

"Thanks for your support," she said. Her eyes brimmed with tears.

After we ate lunch, had coffee and polished off something Darlene called Fluff, I stood up and cleared my throat. "I think it's about time to head over to the hospital, don't you, Shar?"

She nodded.

"Wait. I have a little something for you," Darlene said. She nudged Jon. "You know the one I mean. Can you run into the bedroom and get it?"

He strolled back with a small gift-wrapped box, the kind jewelers use, and handed it to Sharon.

"For me?"

Darlene wagged a finger at Sharon. "Don't open it now. Wait 'til you get settled into the hospital." Her sister took it and slipped it into Sharon's purse.

She made a face. "What if I don't want to wait?"

Darlene and Jon exchanged a glance as if they'd discussed this ahead of time. His look said *I told you so.* "Sis, I thought if you had something to open there, it might not feel so overwhelming. We wanted to do something that would get you through that feeling."

"I get it. Thanks." The sisters hugged. "Be sure to visit

me."

"We will, don't worry."

***

Once on the hospital campus, we checked into the efficiency apartment that would house me while Sharon received her treatment. A consortium of churches had raised funds to provide the nearby complex, specifically for the families of cancer patients to stay during lengthy treatments. It would take only five minutes to walk to the hospital and would save me from having to brave the Houston traffic twice a day. It also saved us the cost of parking all day in the hospital high-rise parking garage.

Next stop, the hospital. While I completed the mountain of paperwork necessary to get the ball rolling, a staff member took Sharon to her room. I walked in and found her stretched out on the bed watching TV. When she saw me, she muted the sound. She already had on a hospital gown. *Here we go again.* With a light touch to my arm, she pushed me away. "I'll be all right for now, Joe. Why don't you go and unpack?"

"Are you sure?"

"Positive. I'll watch some television." She turned up the volume and waved me out. Sharon was not really a television person.

Uncomfortably reassured, I went to the apartment to sanitize the four rooms.

The volunteer staff at the complex had assured me that a person cleaned and sterilized each apartment after the departure of a guest.

"That's all right. I need to do it myself to satisfy the compulsive streak in me." I made a face as if to say 'this is just one of my idiosyncrasies.'

"Well, if you're sure, but we do have a very competent staff that..."

"I know you do." I thanked the woman and closed the door, eager to begin my task. I scrubbed all the floors with a disinfectant soap and applied Lysol to every surface that any human, animal or crawling critter could have touched. I needed to keep my hands busy. The more I thought about the days ahead, the harder I scrubbed.

I sprayed Lysol on everything, even the slats of the mini-blinds. Somewhere in the back of my mind, I felt I was regaining control of our world, even if for just a moment.

But even more than that, I did it because Sharon would be coming to stay in the apartment for a couple of weeks afterward. *We have invested ourselves way too much to have any germ attack her and undo what we've worked so hard to accomplish.* I pointed the Lysol at the doorknob and gave it a good spray as I closed the door behind me. I stood on the steps, aimed the nozzle at my socks and sprayed, then slipped on my shoes.

When I returned to the hospital, Sharon took a gold necklace out of the box. "Honey, honey, honey. *Look.*" The engraving read EXPECT A MIRACLE.

"Can you get the clasp? How many necklaces have you seen like this? I'm going to show it to every doctor and nurse in the hospital and tell them that God has me here to expect a miracle and they are part of it."

I fumbled around to get my size fourteen fingers to close the delicate clasp. "Damn thing." *There.* "Let's see it."

"It's beautiful," Shar murmured, touching it as if it was the Hope Diamond. She walked to the bathroom mirror to admire it. As she settled back in bed, she turned to me and frowned over her glasses. "Now if I can only get you to stop swearing." *That will truly be a miracle.*

I smiled. Truth was, most of my cussing days were behind me. I grew up in a blue-collar neighborhood of row houses in McKees Rocks in Pennsylvania and worked with a hard lot of men in Steel Mills and on summer construction crews for years. This kind of language—and even stronger—made up our core vocabulary. But I'd changed a lot over the years, especially after I met Sharon. "I'm a damn—darn—sight better than I was once upon a time. But thank you for the reminder." I saluted her.

I looked at myself as a diamond in the rough, and my wife, the one who polished me, not just about language, but when it came to manners and clothing as well. I tended to react from my gut. She taught me to slow down and think before I acted. She, like most women knew exactly which clothing went best together. As a result, most of the time, I consulted her before getting dressed for an event or buying anything new to wear. Heck, my friends and relatives even asked her what to get for me sometimes.

The next day Sharon and I met the entire team of specialists who would be working with her case. The lead physician, Dr. Judith Lobo, took time to give an overview of the procedure. Throughout the entire treatment, scores of doctors, interns and nurses would monitor her.

Dr. Lobo turned to me, "Your role in this clinical trial is extremely important. You and your wife are a team here. The more support she receives from you, the better. It won't always be easy. Some spouses don't handle it well."

"No, I'll be fine," I assured her. "Actually, I worked with a home health care service for about six months a couple years back. I dealt with several elderly and critically ill people in my job."

Sharon touched my shoulder. "Honey, God was

preparing you for this time in our life."

We stared at each other. Full of wonder, I said, "I guess He was."

It all fit together how I'd been drawn to that work for His purposes, as Shar would say. After retiring and moving to Erie, I'd wanted a part-time job and that kind of work appealed to me. The one thing that I failed to mention was how emotionally draining it was for me to watch my patients die.

The staff quickly learned about Sharon's aversion to needles. The hospital allowed me to administer the shots in order to kick-start Sharon's body into the production of stem cells. She seemed to have great confidence in my ability to "shoot-her-up." I'd give her two shots a day to speed up the growth of her stem cells for the transplant and would continue giving them to her for the next two weeks.

That morning, doctors and technicians took pains to

explain the details of the necessary med-a-port that would be inserted into her chest below her right clavicle. Their explanation did nothing to assuage Sharon's fears.

Every time she needed to be moved, they brought an attendant with either a gurney or a wheelchair. Transport beds scared us. Wheelchairs weren't as frightening. They simply transported us to tests. Gurneys meant something more serious.

"I'm perfectly capable of walking. I'm discovering no matter which hospital I go to, everyone thinks you're too sick to do anything on your own." She made a face. "But it's kind of fun being pushed in a wheelchair. You never know what United Nations representative you're going to meet next."

A bunch of people from foreign countries pushed her around. She enjoyed talking to anyone from another country with a different accent. Often we played "Twenty

Questions" trying to determine their country of origin. I usually joined in the conversation trying to use the same dialect the attendant did.

Every now and again Sharon would dramatically roll her eyes to stop me. She'd whisper, "Stop making fun of their accent."

"I'm not." I just unconsciously picked up accents well. I'd always had this talent. It didn't matter if the accent were African-American, Southern or Mexican. The way I saw it, I was putting them at ease. I thought that I was pretty good at German and Italian.

A Jamaican-speaking bed attendant took us downstairs to a first-floor room, one that only did insertions of Med-a-ports. Although they didn't drag her kicking and screaming, I could feel the tight grip of her small hand in mine as I held it on the elevator trip down. Shar was seated in a wheelchair, her face pasty-white. She kept pressing her lips together and swallowing, a sure sign she was trying not to cry. She closed her eyes…fighting for control. "It'll be okay, honey." I whispered. *Would it?* I sure as hell hoped so.

This department had it's own doctor, anesthesiologist, pharmacist, medical staff, nurses, and counselors. I guess the counselors were supposed to calm the patient and the patient's worried family. In our case, *I* was the worried family. I began to doubt the need for counselors when they put me into a family waiting room and then forgot where they put me.

I kept constant vigilance with my watch because we had been told that the insertion procedure would just take a little while. One thing I've noticed through all our hospital stays is that the people in charge avoid explaining how "just a little while" translates into seconds, minutes, or hours. I called to the counselor's retreating back, "How long is just a little while? Will I have enough time to drive downtown for a couple of beers?" She never even smiled or responded to my little joke. *Stuffed shirt.*

Five hours later, I continued to sit in the waiting room. No one had come to inform me about the progress or lack of progress they were having with Sharon's procedure. Shifting and readjusting my body did nothing for the flat shape that my backside had assumed. Pins and needles were supposed to be inserted into pincushions and not my rear. I had to get up and walk through a set of double doors to get to the unit's reception desk where I cleared my throat several times before anyone turned to acknowledge my presence.

A woman—the same woman that checked Sharon in for her procedure—looked up, as if to say, "May I help you?" Her question surprised me. I'd been with my wife this morning. I didn't think anyone could miss a big, stocky guy like me but this young woman obviously had.

"I was here with my wife Sharon Belan about five hours ago to have an insertion procedure done and I was wondering if she was finished yet?"

"Your name?"

That was just the start of the inane questions she requested. She asked question after question, without even looking up. She just plunked the information into her computer. After several minutes of wasting my time, I thumped the desk gently with an open palm. When she looked up, I gave her my patented Belan glare. "What is *your* name? Why don't you go in the back and look for her or just make a phone call?"

As I stood there waiting patiently for her response, a female dressed in surgical garb, gloves and facemask walked through the door and announced loud enough for people in the street to hear her, "Mr. Belan, there you are.

We have been looking all over for you. Follow me."

I caught myself just in time and bit back my retort, rolling my eyes instead. By that I meant, *Well, you found me*. I marveled. A couple of years ago, I would have lit into her.

"Your wife's in here," the woman said keeping several steps ahead as if slightly afraid of me. She led me into a large room with about five or six curtained off sections. There reclining on an elevated bed was my beautiful wife with the biggest crooked smile on her face, smiling broadly at me. She even slurred her words as she told me, "Whatever they gave me, I want some more of it." Sharon was not a drinker. She told me how wonderful everyone in the room was and started introducing them. I walked up to the side of the bed and kissed her chastely. I think she liked it. *Just like in our early days in the Great Room.*

"I was getting a little concerned. It took longer than I

thought it would."

Sharon bobbed her head. "They had a few problems. They even had to call someone to complete the procedure." Sharon laughed. Then she looked stricken. "I mean, the doctor knew how to do it, I'm sure, my body just wasn't copper, um, co-oper, helping, them to do it." She gave another big smile as if to say 'my friends are not to blame.'

The attending physician pulled me aside. "Excuse me, sir. We did have some unexpected difficulties. But we resolved them." He handed me a set of instructions regarding the care and cleaning of Sharon's new Med-a-Port.

This time a Filipino attendant magically appeared for the return trip to my wife's room. I did not attempt to copy his accent.

We harvested the stem cells a couple of times over the next two weeks.

The first batch needed time to grow after I started giving the shots. Then doctors permitted Sharon to rest for a few days. When the cells had grown enough to collect them, a short, squat, olive-skinned woman, her straight black hair pulled back in a ponytail, arrived with a wheelchair. "Sher-an Beelan? Vamos … al room de Extraction."

We took the elevator to the second floor. When we exited, I walked alongside the wheelchair. The technician turned left into a room about two thousand square feet. It had three or four extraction machines about the size of two double-wide refrigerator freezers. They were made up of high gauge stainless steel, polished to mirror quality, and looked to me like huge custard machines without the taps for extruding the custard.

I took in the televisions suspended from the ceiling in front of the beds. Near the entrance of the room, I saw what looked like a fifteen-foot gray storage cabinet.

I jabbed my finger in its direction. "What does that hold?"

"About two thousand DVDs and VHS movies," replied a doctor waiting in the room.

The technician pulled the wheelchair alongside the bed and helped Sharon cover up before backing out of the room with the chair.

"Mr. Belan, you and your wife might want to choose a movie. This extraction process will take several hours," advised the attending nurse. She adjusted her bed so that Sharon sat two-thirds of the way, upright. "Are you comfortable?"

"Yes, I'm okay."

The doctor and nurse bustled around getting things set up.

The nurse warned Sharon in advance. "Now, you're

going to feel cold because in order to preserve the stems cells, we have to keep everything at a low temperature. When you feel the cold, just let one of us know and we'll give you a heated blanket. If you're still cold, we'll heat up another blanket in the microwave."

"Okay." Sharon grimaced. She abhorred the cold about as much as she hated needles.

"All the blood will go into this centrifuge. The machine will separate the stem cells from the rest of the blood. After that, the hemoglobin, the white blood cells and all the rest of the blood will be returned to your system," explained the doctor.

"So, it's pretty straightforward?" she asked, matter-of-a-factly.

"Yes, this machine is super-efficient. After we remove the stem cells, we freeze them until it's time to re-insert them into your system. Do you have any questions?"

"In the interim, I'll get the super strong chemo to destroy the cancer cells, is that right?"

"Yes, that's correct."

"When you re-insert the stem cells, they'll fight any stray cancer cell in my body, am I right?"

"Correct, again. You've done your homework."

"Okay, I think I understand and I'm ready."

Her voice sounded quiet but not afraid. As the doctor and nurse prepared for the extraction procedure I sat silently by to lend my support.

Not long into the procedure, Sharon's teeth started chattering. "Brrrrr. I'm freeeezing. I think I'd like a hot blanket." Seconds later, the nurse tucked a heated blanket around her. Right away, we got an assembly line going.

Sharon would say, "Can you give me another blanket, please?"

I'd pick one up from the pile and say, "Warm this one

up." The nurse would hand it off to me. I'd remove the cold blanket and replace it with the new dry, heated one, careful not to bump the arm attached to the machine.

That evening, I kissed Sharon. "You did well, honey. I'm proud of you. Just one more 'harvest' to go next week."

"That's what I call a fast season," Sharon quipped, with a twinkle in her eye. "Harvest. Get it?"

After we collected all the stem cells, we went on to the second phase of the study, what I called the super-chemo treatments. I say "we" because I'm an 'empath,' which means that everything Sharon experienced, I also felt. I got nausea right along with her. For five days straight, Sharon would receive the strongest chemicals ever designed to kill cancer cells. Unfortunately, it would also kill her immunities.

The doctors warned us in advance. "This chemo tends to give the patient adverse side effects—mouth and throat sores. To avoid this, she can suck on ice cubes or popsicles. Hopefully, she won't have to cope much with that on top of everything else. These precautions are very important."

"Honey, I'm worried. I'm not much of an ice-sucker."

"Well, I guess you'd better become one. You like banana and cherry, don't you?"

"Yes, I think I can handle those flavors."

"Say no more." Within twenty minutes, I'd left the hospital and headed to the apartment, picked up a cooler and drove straight to *Food Giant,* a nearby grocery, situated two blocks from the apartment. I scanned the frozen dessert section for popsicles. "Here we go. Cherry." I picked up an entire case. I peered into the glass as I went down the line reading the flavors printed on the brown cartons. I retraced my steps. *No banana.* Finally, I located a stock girl, "Certainly you have banana popsicles, don't you?"

"Let me check in the back, sir."

If they didn't have any, I'd just have to convince Shar to eat more of the cherry. But what if she developed an aversion to one flavor alone? The chemo affected her sense of taste. To be on the safe side, I'd better try my best to find banana.

The stock girl came back beaming. "Here we go, sir. I happened to locate this one lone case of banana popsicles in the corner. It had your name written all over it."

"You mean my wife's name. You're a living doll!" I gave her two thumbs up for her effort and went straight to the cashier, anxious to return to the hospital. At the check-out, I told the bag boy that I did not need help getting the popsicles to my car and loaded into the trunk.

Back at the hospital, doctors permitted me to keep them in the patient lounge freezer.

After the chemotherapy started, I kept busy promoting the popsicles. "Here honey," I urged. "Why don't you have another banana flavored one? You had cherry last time." I was determined to get her to suck enough to prevent her lips, tongue and throat from becoming sore. So, sometimes I had to persuade her that it was for her own good.

That they permitted her to get up and walk with me around the ward astonished me. We'd walk slowly. More often than not, Sharon pushed her portable IV along. I noticed that while the exercise drained her of energy, it got her blood moving. Our first time out, she caught her breath and grunted, "Look, Joe, it's even marked off so we can tell how many miles we walk. The halls were marked off in tenths of a mile. They think of everything here."

"I guess they do." I let them think of everything because I was busy thinking of my wife.

As we came to the fourth day, I noticed how tired Shar looked. She said, "I feel terrible. I so want to make it through this part. Please help me, honey. My *whole* body hurts."

I felt her forehead and reported, "Doctor, she's freezing and burning up sweat at the same time."

A slew of medical personnel put their heads together and discussed the issue. "Mrs. Belan, we'll let you rest for today. Tomorrow, we'll see how you're faring and go on from there."

"Thank you," she said, her voice barely audible. She turned to me and whispered, "This chemo's killing everything but *not* me."

I smiled, grateful for the reprieve. I pressed my lips to her hand. As long as she retained her sense of humor, she'd make it.

She somehow survived the harsh super-chemo treatment and went on to the next phase. Now she faced another critical test, making it through until she was strong enough to receive the stem cells back. Since another patient on the floor was suffering from a virus, the doctors placed her under quarantine. Her room now became an "isolation room" with specially-filtered air to protect her from germs. The air was constantly circulated, drawn out, sanitized, filtered, and then returned to the room at a precise temperature setting.

Doctors described her as hanging somewhere in the fragile state between life and death. A single microbe could undo all the efforts to help her survive. My wife and I had gone through so much together. All she had to do was make it through this time and we'd be home free. I needed to be right with her. Cheering her along with me would be her sister Darlene. She brought her mother-in-law with her. All three of us waited for permission to visit Sharon in her special isolation room.

An attendant instructed us to wash our hands carefully and then showed us what we needed to wear to enter

Sharon's room. It was a bit like preparing for an audience with The Bubble Girl. We donned sterile blue latex gloves. We fit ourselves into puffy, yellow gowns. We even covered our shoes with large yellow booties, and our hair with yellow paper caps. All this just to go in and see Sharon? I couldn't wait to be by her side again, but like this? In these get-ups? "Just like mutant ducklings looking for their mother," I mumbled with a smile.

I entered the room first. "Hey Shar, get a load of these masks. It looks like a duckbill."

She giggled. "You do look like an oversized duck."

"I resemble that remark." I said.

Darlene and June entered the room, slowly, a little uncertain of what to do or how to act.

When I saw the three of us together in the room walking around like a flock of misshapen ducks, I flapped my arms and waddled up to the bed. "Quack, quack."

"You've got *quite* the waddle," Darlene said. She burst out laughing. I swung my behind back and forth as I ventured closer to her. "Quack, quack" I said, with two puffs of air coming from under my mask.

She strutted back and forth across the room to show off her duck waddle to Shar, then turned in a circle and gave her butt a big shake. "Quack, quack," she said back. "Your turn, June," she said to her mother-in-law. "Let's see your best duck imitation."

I thought she might try to get out of it. She was a very dignified lady. But she didn't. She toddled around the room, shuffling her feet and swaying from side-to-side doing the worst rendition of any duck I ever saw. At my guffaw, she came right up to me and gave the shrillest "Quack-quack-quack-quaaack," I ever imagined.

As if by pre-arranged plan, we all began to quack and waddle around the quiet room. "You have the biggest wing span," declared Darlene, laughing.

"But June has the best duck feet," I said, pointing to them. Wide yellow booties shuffled in response, her attempt at the two-step.

"Ladies, follow me," I said and led a procession around the bed, waddling to the best of my ability. I kept a careful distance in the event any spare germ had leaped onto our duckbills. "Spread out … and one-two-three, let's waddle!" I let loose and over-waddled. In fact, we all did.

Sharon tried to lift her head off the pillow but in the end, laid it back down. To my relief, I noticed a small smile and a glimmer of green sparkle in her eyes.

We made such a ruckus that several nurses and interns cruising by stopped in to see what was going on. One of the nurses who peeked in said, "What have we here?"

"Just a roomful of yellow ducks," I said, flapping my arms.

"Quack. Quack," rasped Sharon.

Her voice reminded me that she was still in a precarious condition. It must have taken all her energy to interact with us. Despite wearing such ridiculous costumes and sharing a good laugh, we wouldn't be doing it if she weren't in such delicate health. *Please God, let it go in our favor. Protect this remarkable woman you've put in my life.*

Chapter 12
NEW HOPE

Okay, onward to the next phase. Dr. Lobo briefed us. "It's very clear that the high-dose chemotherapy has physically weakened you. The addition of the stem cells will weaken you even more. When we introduce the stem cells, it will, for lack of a better word, *reboot* your immune system. But in the process, you will experience every single one of the worst influenza symptoms imaginable. It'll take at least fifteen days for your stem cells to become implanted."

Sharon gulped. "I'm ready." She picked up a pad of paper and read some questions off it. "What doesn't kill me is bound to make me stronger, right?" *Great. Who's to say what won't kill her?* Every swear word I knew ran through my mind as I imagined the difficulties Sharon faced.

Damnit. I wish I could control all the variables but we just have to go through them. *I have to help her make that touchdown. Carry the ball whenever I can.*

Unlike removing the stem cells, reinserting them took very little paraphernalia, in fact, only an IV drip. At least we got to stay in Sharon's room for the procedure. Those little droplets we cultivated earlier were the ones that would save her life. It just hit me as weird. If what the doctors said were true, every time a cancer cell showed its ugly face, Shar's new immunities would surround and kill it. I sure hoped so.

On the wall hung an erasable board that you could write on with a board marker. I drew a chart with fifteen numbers on it, and left a space next to the numbers to write or draw something. I wanted to have something to count off the days and to amuse her at the same time. To be honest, I put it up there to amuse myself as well.

The day Sharon's stem cells were reintroduced into her system, she lay in bed. Of course, I sat right by my wife's side. Because the chemotherapy had affected her eyes, she couldn't do anything except possibly watch the television, which we'd turned on earlier.

"What do you want to watch, honey?"

"Oh, whatever. Might as well keep it on that channel."

At the very moment the stem cells started to flow into her, a movie began.

"Joe, look. That's…."

"…John Travolta's *Staying Alive*."

Sharon and I stared at each other and at the drip. She started crying and laughing at the same time. "This is *no* coincidence. It's God telling us He's in control of everything. What a sense of humor." She reached out her arms, as much as you can when you are attached to a drip, anyway. "Goosebumps," she said, pointing to them.

"Me, too," I responded, showing her mine. I swiped at the tears coming to my eyes. I felt as if the wind had knocked me over with the relief of it all. *This trial will give me back my wife.*

When the doctor came in, we told her about the name and timing of the movie. She clapped her hands and touched them to her heart. She smiled, obviously touched by our story, and turned to my wife. She pointed to the drip. "Sharon, today is your new birthday."

Later that day, something else remarkable happened.

We'd been told that you could put the TV weather station in Houston on a film loop and it would be the same, day after boring day. Every now and then Mother Nature threw in a curve ball and pushed through a huge low pressure system that produced angry, dark, roiling clouds, lots of rain and lightning, moving quickly from southwest to northeast and disappearing within an hour of appearing.

That day we observed such a weather phenomena from her fourteenth-story hospital room. The sky grew instantly black. We noticed that all the flags below were standing straight out and flapping like crazy. The most amazing lightning show with the loudest sound effects that either of us had ever heard followed that. Mixed with that was a heavy downpour that reduced our vision from ten miles to a few feet. We couldn't see the buildings right next to us.

As quickly as the storm struck, we watched that weather cell race northeasterly as lightning flowed from sky to ground, bristling with thunderous explosions. Sunshine, and then jagged light burst through the cloud cover and just like a curtain rising on a stage, we saw the rain recede and watched the most beautiful rainbow develop before our eyes. Each band of color stood out clearly from the one next to it.

Since we always looked for signs of hope, we viewed this as "our rainbow." We saw it as a sign from God that this terrible storm of cancer would soon pass over us.

"The movie *Staying Alive* at just the right time and now this incredible storm and rainbow. Joe, how could this stem-cell procedure *not* work?"

It took eight or nine hours to slowly get all of her stem cells back into her body. She shivered like crazy because the hospital kept the stem cells in a cold solution. We repeated the hot blanket assembly line technique throughout. Now came the anxious moments waiting for the flu symptoms to begin.

I saw Sharon clutch the back of her head with her fingers. "My brain is throbbing." She sank back onto the pillow. Her eyes fluttered and closed. She didn't say anything for a minute or two, and I feared that she'd blacked out. But she moved, cupping her eyes and massaging the surrounding area.

"What's wrong with your eyes?" I asked.

"Hmmph? My eyes? Ohhhhhh, it's like I have something sharp poking into the back of my eyeball." She pressed her fingers into her eyelid feeling around. "Like glass. I can't get to it," she muttered.

Here we go. I focused on getting Sharon to eat something. Because this process was going to take up to fifteen days she still needed to eat which gave her something to regurgitate instead of the dry heaves.

The next morning, her red, swollen eyes greeted me. As she blew her nose, I noticed her steel trash bin was filled with soggy tissues.

"Hi huddy," she said, in a stuffed-up voice.

"When did this come on?"

"Biddle of the dight."

I picked up a red marker and next to the second day, I drew a big nose and floating tissue with the word "A-choo" written across it on the erasable board. Shar started to laugh but before long, she brought a hand to her throat as if it hurt her, and had a coughing fit. I thought, "Maybe a popsicle would work."

Take it easy. I felt terrible watching her struggle and rubbed her back in hopes that it would relax her. Instead, she grabbed for the spit bucket. I held her up so she wouldn't lose her balance as she leaned over it. She jerked involuntarily and the contents of her stomach bubbled out of her mouth and dribbled along the outside rim of the bucket.

As I continued to hold her, I felt another wave come over her. Before anything could come out, she threw her head back in the throes of sneezing or coughing or both. A glass-like clear vomit shot across the bed.

Her body trembled but finally regained control. I handed her a tissue. "Blow."

She blew obediently, tapped her foot on the pedal to her metal garbage bin and dropped the dirty tissue inside. I used a warm, wet towel to wipe her face and helped her lie back down. Then I went over to the sink and ran a washcloth under cold water and applied it to her forehead. I folded the cloth in half and pressed it to her neck. This seemed to help her relax a bit. It had been a rough morning so far.

I ached for her, and felt exhausted just watching her suffer. The empty calendar I'd made stared boldly back at me as somehow mocking our efforts. I wondered how we would bear fourteen more days of this.

After several instances of throwing up, Sharon held her stomach and groaned. I turned to the doctor, "It looks to me like she's in terrible pain after throwing up so many times.

Can you not give her something?"

The doctor on duty observed her and consulted with a nurse. "We can give her Tylenol. That might help ease it."

"Hey, doc, have a heart. Can't you give her something stronger, say along the lines of Oxycodone or Hydrocodone?"

He shook his head and walked away from us. I thought he had gone to consult another doctor or nurse on the situation but as he exited the room, I finally realized the subject was closed. He hadn't even bothered to give an explanation. *What if it were your wife? Yeah, what if?*

I took a deep breath. *We'll make it through this, too.* But try as I might, it still rankled me. That evening in the apartment, I wondered what he thought of my request. He'd probably seen this response many times throughout the clinical trials and found her responses typical of what one went through. Nothing out of the ordinary that would call for special treatment. But even so, why didn't he explain that to me? Would I have bought it if he had? While she might have been just another patient to him, I was watching the love of my life puke out her guts, and then some. I closed my eyes and tried to rest.

I entered the room the next morning. "Do we have any new symptoms today?" I teased.

"Why yes, as a matter of fact, we do. We have muscle pain along with backaches."

"Let me at them," I said, "I give a great body massage. I won't even charge."

She turned over on her stomach and I took my time, lovingly kneading and caressing the afflicted muscles, praying my ministrations made a difference. I couldn't help but notice how thin her limbs had become, so I made sure that I massaged her gently. Not the best of times, but I sure loved the feeling of being connected to her through our touch.

"Perfect," she said forty-five minutes later. "If I can just get that two or three more times today, I'll be good to go."

"Glad to oblige. How about something to eat? It's about eleven o'clock."

"I can't. My stomach's cramping up again." She touched a hand to her abdomen and took a deep breath and exhaled. "Let's see what's on TV," she said brightly.

I flipped it on. "I keep expecting to see surrender etched on your beautiful face but all I ever see is that 'Stark' look of determination."

She giggled. "Good pun. Too bad I married a Belan and changed my name."

A couple of days later, I sat beside her bed. "Joe, how about reading me some more of Morrie's book."

I was reading her *Tuesdays With Morrie* aloud. Hearing

my voice soothed her, she said. She liked to lie there with her eyes closed and picture the old man sharing his ideas with his former student. I opened the book, pulled up a chair near the bed and began.

I was into the second page, when Shar looked up with a stricken look. "Oh. My. God. I gotta get to the toilet *now*," she said urgently. "Joe, help me up." I tossed the book aside and jumped up to aid her. We raced to undo her wires and the tubes that held her down. "Joe, hurry, *Joe*." Free at last, she sprinted to the toilet, about five feet away.

Is she going to make it? Whew. That was close.

"Joe."

I raced to the bathroom and swung open the partially-closed door. *Oh no.* I found her clutching the sink, sobbing. I surveyed the room, and my heart went out to her. The second urge wound up splattering the wall, the toilet, and a major portion of her bed clothing.

"I can stand anything, any pain, any vomiting. I don't even mind that this happened. But I can't stand for *you* to see me like this," she said again and again through her tears.

"Sharon Belan, you're my *sunshine*. Don't be embarrassed. There's no reason. There is *nothing* I wouldn't do for you. Let's get you cleaned up."

"I know, but I don't want you to *see* me this way." The tears seemed to clog her throat, and her shoulders drooped as she shook her head.

"Let's get you out of those pajamas and washed up," I repeated. "Sharon, I *love* you. We're in this together, remember?" We took off her pajamas. "How about if you wear a nightgown?" I suggested. "It might be easier."

She nodded and I helped her back into bed. I filled a bucket with water and some disinfectant soap and cleaned up the bathroom in case Sharon needed to use it again soon immediately. While I was doing that, she pressed the button for the nurse to report what had happened. Within seconds the nurse arrived. Soon, an orderly came to go over what I'd already done. Crazy, but hospitals have their rules. *That's just what I did with the apartment.* I bagged everything up to take home to wash. Her bed clothes would be washed, rinsed, and sanitized twice.

Upon learning of Sharon's accident, the nurses brought in a port-a-john that could be placed conveniently next to the bed. The distance from the toilet wasn't the problem. She had so many tubes and wires attached to her that by the time she got untangled, sometimes she just couldn't make it.

I wondered why it *didn't* bother me more. I guess as Shar said, God prepared me a long time ago when I did that stint at the senior care facility. Cleaning up after bodily functions became routine. Besides, this is *Sharon,* the love of my life. I would do that and much more for her.

"According to our wedding vows," I said, tenderly touching her cheek, "we promised to care for each other. What just happened falls in the sickness clause of our marriage contract, and I'm duty bound," I gently teased.

Nothing that I could do or say assuaged her feeling of embarrassment.

That night back in the apartment, I washed the soiled clothing. As I threw them in the dryer, I took out my Sudoku puzzles. Focusing my energy on these puzzles kept me from replaying what had gone on in the hospital on any given day. It's not that I didn't care or feel anything. It's that I didn't want to dwell on what we were going through. I needed to keep my mind fresh for Sharon. Perhaps later, when we were safely past these challenges, I'd have the luxury of recalling our day-to-day struggles—but not here and not now.

Almost in reverse order the symptoms began to disappear. The last to go were the headaches. One morning she awoke in bed with that rosy glow on her cheeks, and that famous Sharon Belan smile punctuated with those twinkling eyes, and I knew that we were through the worst of it.

On the erasable board next to the number eight, I drew a big smiley face with a bedpan flying out of the window.

All the doctors and nurses came to celebrate with us. Our football team analogy came to mind. "Shar, remember how we said you'd get through this with your teammates. You're making your touchdown, after all. You ran with the ball down that muddy…"

"Barf-covered…" she added, with a grin.

"…field."

"I haven't made that touchdown yet. We have to wait to see if trial succeeded," she reminded. She surprised me, like she always did as she called her "team" together and gave another explanation.

"God told me to read Joshua while I was in Houston. It's all about battle after battle to win the Promised Land. God told Joshua to rely on Him, promising that He would fight the battles and win the victory. I was praying every day, telling God that I knew it was His battle. I claimed His victory over ovarian cancer and asked Him to respond through me. I asked Him to get me through these symptoms not in fifteen days, not in twelve days, but in *eight* days. Today is the eighth day. God fulfilled my heart's desire." Sharon's eyes were alight with excitement and praise.

The hospital faculty and staff listened respectfully as she spoke, smiling and congratulating us. Yes, praising God, too. I kept shaking my head in wonder. For a man who never ran out of words, I certainly couldn't put into words the relief I felt.

Dr. Lobo came in and wrapped her fine surgeon's arms around my wife. "This is as fast as we've ever seen any patient's stem cells become engrafted. *Eight days.* That's a record. Seventy-five percent of any battle like this is attitude. You've consistently demonstrated the power of the positive throughout this very difficult trial."

"It's not *me*. It's God," my wife emphasized, yet again.

The way all the doctors, nurses and staff cheered, you'd have thought that this good news had happened to them. In a way, I guess, it did. Sharon touched everyone with her faith and optimism. I couldn't believe if everything worked out, we'd have our life back, and be living out the "to have and to hold" part of our marriage vows again.

After Sharon was discharged, I took her to the apartment where we stayed for the next two weeks. Dr. Lobo wanted us nearby in the event of an unforeseen emergency. I continued to keep the apartment sanitized and immaculate. I even continued to spray even the doorknobs and my shoes so Sharon would not fall prey to a single germ—not after all we had gone though.

At the dinner table that night, she bubbled over with excitement. "Joe, can you believe that we shared our faith with people from all over the world here in Houston, doctors and nurses who came from the Philippines, Vietnam, Colombia and Nigeria and all sorts of places? Guess what else? They believed in Jesus and played a part in God's plan for us."

"We sure did. That's why I call you Shar'. You're always *sharing* The Good News with everyone you meet. You came in expecting a miracle—and *received* it."

She touched the necklace that she never took off, even to shower. As I listened to my wife talk, I thought about how she was changing the way I viewed adversity. In facing it, I thought most people behaved like I did. I'd puff myself up, make loud aggressive noises, shout, curse, threaten and intimidate anyone who crossed me.

She did none of these things. Instead, when she was deeply upset, she'd retreat deep inside herself, and pray. If I made her angry, she'd stare straight ahead, cross her arms and keep silent. Her silence unnerved me because it could go on interminably.

When faced with adversity like this cancer, she reached out to those closest to her for support and gathered friendships like bunches of flowers along the way— doctors, nurses and even other patients. She won them over with her optimism and sweet nature. More often than not, she turned to the Bible and prayed to God, whom she called The Great Healing Physician.

Maybe she had something there. Maybe I needed to think more about how faith operated. I spent my whole life pitching myself against foes, and winning. This damn cancer would not toe the line. In fact, it constantly bucked against us, as if it took deliberate joy in besting foes. What if I did give it over completely to God? Was this a test? Would He give us the cure then? *Is He waiting on me?*

The thought scared the hell out of me.

Chapter 13
RESULTS OF CLINICAL TRIAL

As it drew nearer to the time to return to M.D. Anderson Hospital for the third time, the tension grew stronger. A lot was riding on the outcome of our visit to the doctor.. After several follow-up tests, Sharon and I would meet with her team to discover the results of the autologous stem cell replacement planted nearly a year ago.

We talked about it again the night before we left. I said, "I can't wait to find out what the doctors tell us. You'll see. Our lives are going to turn around."

"Oh, honey, I hope so. I don't know if I can go through all that again."

"I know. What you went through…my God! You suffered through the world's worst case of the flu I've ever seen as your body fought the cancer off. My poor baby…" I tucked in the covers tightly around Sharon's body, unconsciously trying to protect her from any other pain and suffering. "But it'll be worth it when we find positive results to the surgery, won't it?" I could hardly wait for that moment to come.

"Oh, Sweetheart, a thousand times yes!"

We focused on the positive. But in thoughts that we never voiced out loud, we both acknowledged the possibility that the surgery might not lead to a cure. In many ways, it was like walking along the beach together with the waves lapping at our feet. All we wanted was to move forward, but with a tug here and a pull there, we were constantly reminded that something stronger could stop us in our tracks and keep us from getting where we wanted to go. We tried to ignore whatever got in our way, whatever stopped us from moving forward. But we both knew that it wasn't possible to control nature.

So far, though, our approach seemed to be working.

Now we'd know for sure. Sharon was preparing herself to

go through a series of exams to determine whether or not

the stem cell procedure had worked. From what the doctors

told us so far, we had high hopes. We only needed the

pathologist and oncologist's confirmation to set our final

fears at rest and confirm what we believed—the treatment

had worked. Soon, Sharon would learn that she is cancer-

free … forever.

"Can you believe M.D. Anderson is located right here

in the US? All we have to do is hop in the car and take a

drive to get there."

"I love that. Another road trip for me. We can visit our

favorite places, and seek out new ones." Sharon clapped

her hands in glee.

I looked at her in amazement. Many women would

have moaned and groaned about the inconvenience of the

drive or fretted about why they had to travel there at all. Not her. Even in this dire situation, she looked for joy in her life. Wow!

As I lay there curled up to my wife feeling like the luckiest man alive, I remembered the first conversation we ever had about travel.

***

Edinboro, 1995

Though I never dreamed Sharon and I would meet up again after Gettysburg, one "hello" led to another and nine hours later, we continued our impromptu date at my friend Mary Sue's place.

We'd been told to make ourselves comfortable so I poked around inside the house, looking for a more private place to talk. "Hey, no one's in the living room. Why don't we have a seat here?" With a grand gesture, I motioned for her to sit down. "An empty couch, great food, what more could we ask for?" I took Sharon's Coke and plate until she could get situated.

"Thanks, Joe."

I couldn't think of a better place to be than next to this wonderful lady.

She suddenly leaned forward, eyes all earnest. "Joe, do you like to travel?"

"You know what? I've been really fortunate in that I've been able to travel to every state in the continental US. Why do you ask?"

"I've dreamed of traveling to new places. Florida. Alaska. Out West." Sharon pummeled a red throw pillow in her passion. "Anywhere in the US."

"Whoa! What's holding you back? Teachers get the whole summer off…"

"Hmph! It's not that easy." She covered her eyes in frustration as she groped for the words to explain. "I was married to…I mean, he never wanted to…we couldn't go *anywhere* far. Uh, he *had* to be back by nightfall to sleep in his own bed, he said. He just, just didn't … like to travel. We rushed here and there—never could enjoy the journey." I didn't know what to say.

A short silence followed. "I guess you've been to the Ocean?" At my nod, she said, "What's it like?"

"What? You haven't been to the ocean?" I was shocked. I thought everyone had seen the ocean—any of them—at least once.

"Nope. Not even close."

"Well, the water sprays so high. It would hit you, ah, at your belly button," I lightly tapped it through her T-shirt. Sharon took my hand and held it for a second. "…or maybe at your waist. The water feels soft and sudsy, depending on where you are, almost like bathwater. But if the salt gets into a cut, watch out! Oooh. And sometimes it gets in your mouth and tastes so salty. It burns if you swallow it— makes me cough my head off. You can see all the way to the horizon."

Sharon pressed her hands together. "Oh, I can just imagine it! I simply must go someday. Someday…"

"There's a really cold, rocky coast in Oregon…" She held on to my words as if they were precious stones, and she savored every detail.

For a while silence reigned.

"This is so cozy." Sharon smoothed out the red cushion now on her lap. "Just the two of us."

"It is." For just a moment, I felt tongue-tied.

***

I started to remind Sharon of that time, but as I looked down at her, I saw that her breathing had become regular. I watched her sleep, marveling that our lives had intersected that day six years ago. *Here we lay, side-by-side, husband and wife, ready to take on the world together.* I tenderly kissed her forehead and cuddled up next to her, yawning. *By God, I'll make sure this trip is everything she wants it to be.*

We set out for Houston as we did every other trip. We brought along our favorite CDs and placed one in the slot. As the garage door closed behind us and we pulled out of the driveway, we repeated our now famous line, "We're off on another excellent Sharon and Joe adventure!"

She took my hand and squeezed it. "Joe, I'm so glad you're with me on this adventure. I need you."

"I'm here, Babe. We're going down these roads together."

We decided to go to Houston via Cleveland, Cincinnati, Memphis and Arkadelphia. Every time we drove through Arkadelphia, we laughed.

The teacher in her came out now. "Honey, that's so crazy. The settlers must have been confused about where they were. Was it Arkansas or Philadelphia?"

"Well, it's like a horse of a different color—or something like that." For some reason, that also struck us funny. We felt really good. I looked over at her and she looked back, and we burst out laughing.

She suddenly reached into the back seat. "The camera! Joe, you remembered it, didn't you? Did you charge it before we left?"

"Yes, I did."

"Good." She turned around and visibly relaxed. "I'm sure we'll have lots of photo ops this trip. I'd just die if we forgot the camera. We'd have to go back. If I can capture some interesting shots then I'll have something to work with when I paint my landscapes."

"Don't worry. I also brought the charger, along with every other charger we'll ever need, even the one to our electric toothbrushes. I made a list. You'll find plenty of unusual trees, clouds, and rocks to photograph."

Since we'd traveled to Houston a couple of times earlier, it turned out to be a trip of re-discovery. Anytime she wanted me to pull over, I did, and she'd take a bunch of photos. I even drove at the speed limit. We stopped to gas up but also stopped just to take breaks and look around the quaint small towns that caught our fancy. We left plenty of time for these side excursions. *I'm getting pretty good at taking time out to enjoy the journey.*

We also had many uninterrupted one-on-one conversations about everything except cancer during our drive to Houston. Maybe we didn't want to ruin the mood by introducing that topic. Maybe it was too delicate a topic to broach. Who knows? Perhaps we simply tiptoed around it because so much rested on the outcome. For whatever reason, we left it alone on that trip.

Sharon tapped the button to start up the CD player again. Our disk had some songs from Koinonia, a men's spiritual retreat. I didn't attend church regularly until after we married. And it wasn't until I attended Koinonia that the songs on this CD meant anything to me.

Sharon tapped my knee. "Honey, isn't this song beautiful? It just makes me feel good."

"Me, too. I sang this song with fifty men at Koinonia."

As I looked over at Sharon, I realized how much my life had changed as a result of her being in my life. She had nudged me into a deeper relationship with God. I took my hand off the wheel and caressed her leg for a moment. "Thank you, Babe."

She gave me a curious look. "For what?"

"Just for being who you are."

She smiled over at me and blew me a kiss. "Right back at you."

My cell phone rang again. We'd both been getting calls throughout the trip from friends and relatives checking on us. Everyone knew how important the results from M.D. Anderson would be. I held my hand over the receiver and mouthed to Sharon, "It's Jon and Bev Franz."

"The epitome of 'inquiring minds want to know,'" Sharon whispered, her eyes crinkling. They were our dearest friends.

"We're holding up fine," I said in response to Jon's question.

I put him on speaker phone so we could all talk. The music we had on the CD caught their attention. "What's that song you have playing in the car?" Bev asked.

"It's *Shine, Jesus, Shine,* our traveling song."

Sharon called out, "We always launch our excellent adventures with this song, and we play it again and again." We sang a few lines into the cell phone to Bev and Jon. Finally, we lowered the volume and talked to them about her upcoming appointment.

"The doctor's going to have good news for Sharon, I'm certain," Bev reassured us at the end of our conversation.

"We sure hope so." I looked over at my wife and saw the hope in her eyes. We promised to keep them posted and rang off. "They'll call us a couple more times today." I laughed, but glad to have so much support.

As on the preceding trips, we stopped at Sharon's sister's place on the outskirts of the city. This time we spent the night.

The next morning, I woke up early. Today would be a big day for us, and I just couldn't sleep. "Good morning,

Sunshine. We need to leave early to avoid traffic. We can park and go for a walk in the amusement park near the hospital here."

"That's a good idea. I could hardly sleep last night."

"I know. Same here." I wish I could have erased the dark circles under her eyes. I would have moved the sun and moon for her, if I could have. She knew that.

I closed the door behind us, admiring how, even at five in the morning, how put-together Sharon looked in a pretty blue sweater and slacks. Yet somehow she looked young and vulnerable right then. I wished that the meeting with the oncologist were already behind us and that we could celebrate. But that would happen soon enough. We hoped.

We wandered through the park by the hospital. "I could be golfing now," I joked as we caught dim glimpses of the golf course through the trees.

"You and your golfing." Sharon snuggled closer to me.

I drew her hand up to my lips and brushed a kiss across it.

"Golfing doesn't always leave me with the best of memories." I thought of the golf outing at Crabapple Golf Course when we first found out about Sharon's cancer. "I don't want to be anywhere else except with you at this moment."

"I can think of one really great memory that has to do with a bunch of golf courses." Sharon said with a sly smile.

I knew exactly what she was referring to—the day of many surprises.

Erie, 1999

In the spring of our fourth year when we were still dating long-distance, Sharon had planned a special day for us.

She demanded I go for a ride with her. When I tried to wheedle where we'd go out of her, she only gave me a mysterious smile. "It's a surprise." She pulled me up out of my chair where I was reading the newspaper. "Come on."

Sharon was acting a little strange. But I got a kick out of her surprises. *What does she have up her sleeve now?* I took my keys off the hook. "Your car or mine?"

"Ha! Ha! Mine this time."

I groaned and hung up my car keys again. Squeezing my 6'6" frame into her little tan Honda took effort but once inside with the seat pushed back, I could stretch out my legs and have enough head room to wear my hat.

She looked over at me, excitement in her eyes. "Buckle up, Buckaroo Bonzai. We are traveling to where no man has gone before."

I stared at her. *Had she gone loco?* She definitely had something out-of-the-ordinary in mind. But what?

"Well?" she prompted.

After buckling up, I slid a CD in the player. Before the music started, we both shouted on cue, "Another excellent

Sharon and Joe adventure!"

Sharon batted her eyes. "Do you remember telling me that there weren't any golf courses in Erie? Well, I'm going to show you more golf courses than you can shake a golf club at."

She must have scoured the phone book to find every golf course in the area because we made a day out of it. We even rode by a couple of country clubs on the way back. She glanced my way and smiled. "We can't afford for you to play there."

We? "You never know. I just might get to be friends with one of your former boyfriends. Chances are he'd invite me to play at the *Kahkwa* with him…"

"None of my former boyfriends ever played golf." Then, just like Edith Ann, the character of a little girl rocking in an oversized rocking chair on *Saturday Night Live*, she gave me a very unladylike raspberry.

Laughter escaped me. "I love this banter that we have. We've gotten to know each other so well, and we aren't even married yet."

"Yet? You said 'Yet.' Is that your way of proposing?"

Her response caught me off guard. I *had* been thinking of proposing. But I hadn't found the appropriate venue to give an event of such magnitude the justice it deserved. I didn't want to be pushed so I snapped, "We gotta talk about a lot of other stuff first."

The half-smile on her face disappeared. The playful air between us instantly evaporated. *When she took me to all those golf courses, was she trying to convince me to move to Erie? Did she want me to propose today? How long had she been waiting? I hope she still wants to marry me. Damn. Did I know how to stick my foot in my mouth or what!*

"Hell, if I knew—" I cut myself off. *Why get into it?*

We rode the rest of the way home in awkward silence. *Way to kill a mood, Joe!* Once home, I opened the back door. A whiff of this morning's cinnamon toast and cold coffee on the stove lingered in the air. As she stepped into the dark kitchen, she reached for the light switch. But I turned her around and made a split-second decision. Since she was on the elevated step, we stood face-to-face. Placing my hands around her slender waist, I looked into her green eyes and whispered, "Will you marry me?"

She blinked and said without missing a beat, "If that's your way of trying to make up and get me into bed, the answer is 'no.'"

I took her into my arms and we dissolved into laughter. I knew in my heart her 'no' actually meant a resounding 'yes.'

We sealed our words with a long, relieved kiss. Our long-distance dating had come to an end.

"Ah….you're still trying to get me into bed every free moment you can! What am I going to do with you?"

I twirled her in a circle, "Guess you're stuck with me."

She paused. "I'm glad I am. You know, Joe, remember how you used to joke about making an honest woman out of me?"

I nodded as we began to walk again. "Mm-hm."

"You weren't too far off the mark."

I stared at her. "What do you mean?"

"Well, as I grew as a Christian, I started to look at my life. I wanted to obey *all* of God's commandments, not just the ones that were easy. That area was one I hadn't turned over to him."

This was news. "I never knew you felt that way."

She looked down at her wedding ring. "Well, let's just say that God was speaking to me about it. I'm glad we got married when we did. It's a beautiful thing and part of His plan … in marriage. I felt much better about us."

I touched the ring, tentatively. "I wish you'd said something. I'd have married you sooner."

She leaned her head on my shoulder. "I know. I guess we had to do some growing."

The first rays of sunlight shimmered through the dim branches of the trees that held lacy appendages of Spanish moss dangling down, reflecting glimmers of the sun's rays. As we walked around the park, she pointed to them. "We beat the sun this morning. It's just now waking up." I took her in my arms and we simply stood for a few minutes, taking in this natural blessing that God gave to calm us on this anxious morning. I smoothed her hair. *Everything is going to be all right. This whole fight for your survival will be over with soon.* Even the park was alive with hope.

As we moved forward, again, she pointed out the beauty that surrounded us, this time the mist that hung about a foot off the ground. Our feet seemed to disappear into that shrouded precipitation. Again, thoughts came to me. This time I recalled the early morning I dropped her off at her room in Gettysburg after we danced that first time together at the workshop. That morning had been foggy as well. How history repeats itself. A lump formed in my throat and I pulled her closer, resting my chin on the top of her head.

How precious this time together is…

Another even more beautiful moment waltzed into our morning. My cell phone rang. It was Bev and Jon. In turn, they wished us good morning. We laughed and thanked them for thinking of us. Jon took the phone then. "Listen up, guys. From our hearts to yours…"

We looked at each other. What was Jon up to?

Suddenly, a loud chorus of voices sounded through the phone, singing *Shine Jesus Shine.* As we stood in the park at that moment, our hearts overflowed with His love. Sun rays shone through that early morning darkness—a tangible outpouring of God's love to us, His beautiful promise as the sky began to lighten.

We had been walking in darkness as we coped with Sharon's cancer over the past year or so. Yet His love and His light had penetrated through. He had guided us through the dark days. When we came to the part of the song about truth setting us free, we stared at each other, thinking of the meeting that lay ahead. What truth was God preparing us for this very afternoon? We gathered renewed strength and hope.

The tears flowed down our faces as we clung to each other, the mist swirling at our feet. We did feel God's presence with us.

We held the phone between us and continued to listen to the church sing to us. Our voices joined theirs on the phone as we rocked back and forth in place, the tears clogging our throats effectively silencing our singing. We sounded triumphant, and joy filled us. What an awesome connection to our Christian brothers and sisters back home and to God reaching out to us. In just those few minutes it took to sing the song, the morning rays brightened, from glimmering to flooding through the trees. We had no doubt that God was speaking to us directly and touching our hearts with the very thing that would impact us. The words infused us with courage to face the meeting and the day ahead.

As the song finished, Bev came on the line. "If you haven't guessed already, we are on speaker phone. That was about two hundred and fifty of us from Summit United Methodist Church. We felt God wanted us to share that song with you this morning."

"It was perfect, and exactly what we needed to hear."

Sharon could hardly speak through her tears. "We thank you more than words can say for this beautiful moment."

Sharon ended the call and turned to me. I brushed her tears away as she brushed mine away. "I can't believe they did that. We'll never forget this song, for sure now, will we?"

"No, we won't." She leaned against me, a smile of peace on her face. "I am ready to face the news."

"Me, too. What a sign from God. The news is going to be good, babe." I kissed her on those words. We felt lighthearted as we walked around the park. A couple of hours later, the smell of hot dogs grilling on a spit reached us. "Want one?"

"Do you even need to ask?"

I yawned. "That sounds great to me, too, and I'll take another cup of coffee. Keep your eye open for a vendor."

We idly explored the amusement park until late

morning. It turned out to be the perfect release for our emotions. Suddenly, we felt an unexpected cold breeze. We stopped walking for a minute and shivered in surprise. Sharon buttoned up her sweater. *Where did that come from?* The break in weather reminded me that we had not driven halfway across the country simply to stroll through an amusement park.

I glanced over at her. "It's time, honey. We need to head over to the hospital."

Sharon squared her shoulders. "Ready."

We took the elevator and walked down the now-familiar hallway to our oncology wing to meet with key members of Sharon's team. I knocked on the door and the oncologist's assistant, Dr. Rose, opened it. Dr. Lobo, head oncologist, waved us in and gestured toward the brown leather chairs situated directly in front of her desk.

As we all waited for the rest of Sharon's team to arrive,

we made small talk about the weather, our appetites, and the trip to Houston. The Patient Advocate and another assistant slipped through the door and took a seat.

We turned expectantly toward Dr. Lobo. She shuffled some papers, looked down at her notes and avoided our eyes. Dr. Rose came over and took Sharon's hand. I scooted my chair closer to my wife. But still no one said anything. Sharon and I looked at each other uneasily. I read confusion and doubt in her eyes, which mirrored my own. I clasped her free hand in my own. *Dear God...*

We researched Dr. Lobo and M.D. Anderson extensively before we started the treatment. One of the five best ovarian cancer oncologists in the country, Dr. Lobo inspired trust. Warm, positive, knowledgeable and up-front with us every step of the way, we felt we made the best choice possible when we chose her to work with Sharon.

But now the silence unnerved me. My heart

thumped…

Finally, Dr. Lobo spoke. Her gaze went to Sharon. She took a deep breath and launched into the feedback. "I hate to tell you this, Sharon. I wish I had better news…"

I fixated on Dr. Rose's ministrations to my wife. *No! No! Don't say it!*

"…The procedure was not successful."

My head slowly turned toward Dr. Lobo. *Had I heard her correctly?*

With Dr. Rose still holding her hand, my wife twisted toward me and buried her face in my chest. I stroked her hair, helplessly.

Dr. Lobo held the results of the tests in her hand. She tapped the paper as she spoke. Her voice broke down. "I don't understand it myself. This is so unexpected. The signs…every sign along the way pointed to very positive results." She stopped to gather her professionalism about her. All the while, the tears slid down her face. "Sharon, we monitored you for nearly a year. The experts on our team believed that the stem cells had implanted. Remember how quickly you responded to the chemotherapy. I'm so, so … sorry but the results are conclusive. It's back, stronger than ever."

Her tears set off a chain reaction. Sharon and the rest of the team, all female, began to sob. Then it happened. Yes, big guy that I am, I lost it, too. Loud blubbery sobs tore through me.

All the hope that we had harbored was crushed.

I, the stalwart knight, could do *nothing*.

My thoughts were reeling. *Didn't we just have the best morning of our life? Hadn't we seen the clearest rainbow we ever saw right during the stem-cell implant? What about the movie, Staying Alive? Had we come into this with unrealistic expectations? Where did the loving God who promised He'd never leave run off to?*

We all got caught up in the grip of grief for a short time.

"Oh, *honey.*" I kneeled on the floor and took her in my arms. "Shh. Shhhh. Shhhh" I held on for dear life as I lay my head on top of hers. We stayed like that, locked in our grief until my anger took over.

With nervous energy, I leaped up. "Clemente said with that smug smile of his, 'We got it all!' And then everyone here, was just *wowed* by her response to the stem-cell implant... How can today's news contradict all that?"

Sharon tugged on my arm. Her look said, *Don't blame the doctors. It's not their fault.*

I forced myself to sit back down. Then it burst out of me. "What ... what does this mean? What are our choices? Another chemo cocktail? What are we looking at here?"

Sharon gave a slight shake of her head. I knew that

look, too. *Don't be confrontational.*

Dr. Lobo faced me. "Joe, there are a few options. But they're long shots…"

I paced in the small room. *Claustrophobic.* "Will she have … are we talking more hospitals? What?" *Is this it? And now just wait for the end to come?* "Help me—help us —understand why this didn't work!"

Sharon sat up and fumbled with a small notebook and pen. "Joe…" She ducked her head at me. I guess that meant to *sit down.* I did so, again, with effort. She flipped the pages back and forth, trying to focus on the questions she'd written in advance.

Dr. Lobo walked around her desk and hugged Sharon. "How about if we all take a deep breath, shall we? We can talk about your options in a few minutes." She handed some tissues to Sharon, took some herself and passed the box to me.

She anticipated Sharon's questions as she eyed the notebook. First, she reassured her. "You are in our system and, of course, we will include you in any future clinical test trials. Why it didn't work, I have no idea. It's an anomaly. Who can say in the end why a body doesn't fight off bad cells?"

Sharon rolled the pen between her hands. "It was too good to be true, I guess." She sighed and began asking the questions we never thought would see the light of day.

"What kind of tests will I have now?"

"Is there anything else you can do for me?"

"What are my chances?"

As she asked the last question, a thought slapped me in the face. One of the many doctors we met along our journey—not sure which one—warned, 'It's essential to successfully treat the cancer the first time because if it comes back, eighty-five percent of the time, it comes back to stay.' *And if it stays, does that mean Sharon won't?*

I loosened my shirt collar that all of a sudden seemed too tight. *Wait! I missed it. How did Dr. Lobo respond to Sharon's question? What ARE her chances?*

The rest of the meeting went by in a blur. I don't know how we got through the crushing disappointment. I don't think any of these professionals get comfortable in delivering the kind of news we received. It's almost as if they're delivering a death sentence. Well, the truth is, they *were.*

Seeing the 'professionals' break down, I suddenly understood how my wife affected them. They had become personally involved. You couldn't find a braver or more positive patient. She'd celebrated every little gain with the staff, and bore the difficulties with courage. They went out of their way to visit her hospital room. Now they, too, had to face this loss.

I didn't know exactly what was going on in Sharon's mind that afternoon but all I could hear was Dr. Lobo's words playing like a broken record in my head. *The cancer is back, stronger than ever.*

We went straight to the parking garage, had no desire to see any more of the park or a single square inch of M.D. Anderson. We wanted to go home. We'd been gone far too long. *Home. Safe. In our own personal space.*

We started the long trip back from Houston in stoic silence. Our cell phones didn't even ring. *Did our friends and family and everyone who supported us now have a sixth sense about the results?*

In the silence, my mind wandered.

I could take any Steelers' loss at the Superbowl. We'd always have next year.

This was more like a loss at the World Series. Of course, much worse. Huh! The World Series of Joe and

Sharon's life ... we'd reached the bottom of the 9th in Game Seven of our World Series. Tied—three wins, three losses. The games had been up and down. Exhilarating victories followed by gut-tearing losses. But it finally looked like the crowning triumph and the trophy, a cancer-free life for Sharon! Team Anderson put in our Stem-cell ace relief pitcher to shut 'em down 1-2-3. All the fans were up on their feet in the stands screaming, "Go! Go! GO!" It looked like the perfect mix, great unhittable pitches again and again when suddenly from out of nowhere, Team Cancer knocked the pitcher out of the box!

What happened next would be talked about around the water cooler for several days...they blasted the ball out of the park. All the team's fans rushed the field and overtook it in celebration. The only problem—the team favored to lose, won. Game over. That was the way I felt, really, the way we *all* felt. We thought our ace pitcher was indomitable. We put all our faith in the stem-cell procedure and it let us down.

What would stop Team Cancer from loading the bases —and smacking the grand slam?

What did we have left to do? *A big fat nothing.*

Well, almost nothing. We'd get more chemo at the Cancer center in Erie. We'd put in our second and third string pitchers. They might surprise us, but would they ever lead us to another Joe and Sharon World Series?

What did that beautiful song *Shine, Jesus, Shine* just as the sun was coming up through the trees mean? Why did God give us that comfort if all He planned to do later was to hurtle us to the depths of despair and prove none of it meant anything?

Why, God? Why? What was the big idea of showing us that damn rainbow the first time we came to M.D.

Anderson, huh? You got both our hopes up. You know that because You know everything! We took it as an early sign of hope. Sharon called it a "reaffirmation" that You would lift her out of this deep valley, but instead You threw her deeper into it! How could you do that?

A driver honked his horn as it sped past me, and I steered the car away from the no passing center line. *You've got to drive safely, Joe. You'll be no help to Sharon otherwise.*

I felt depression lunge onto my shoulder. It was as if it beat at me, swinging with all its might. Somehow desperation fought back. I wanted to bargain with God. *Just give me Sharon. One. Small. Determined. Woman. My wife. I'll do whatever You want me to do. Just don't take Sharon away. You can't bargain with God.*

What could we have done differently? I went back and forth in my mind, wanting to blame someone. It had to be *someone's* fault.

When the big invincible Dr. Clemente with his ninety-eight percent patient success rate looked at the pathologist's report right after the operation, he declared, "We got it all." What if he didn't?

Or, what if the *pathologist* screwed up? Could he have misread the cancer slides? Maybe he was too tired. It happens. The procedure lasted for six hours. Sharon didn't return from the recovery room until after 2:00 am. They got out of surgery so late. The surgeon wanted to have the pathologist's report by 9:00 am. In his rush, maybe he missed something.

I was so caught up in her post-operation well-being that I didn't even begin to question when the doctor, sounding so very full of himself, said, 'No cancer cells at all.' Then to err on the side of caution, he suggested, 'I'll have Sharon take three rounds of chemotherapy, to be on the safe side.'

I smoldered with fury. The cancer came back 'stronger than ever' because some tired SOB read Sharon's lab reports wrong. And the doctor didn't get it all. Or maybe Sharon needed more chemo.

I went back and forth between rational and irrational thought. Cancer took its toll on people, and sometimes it won. As much as we wanted to think practitioners or anyone in the medical field had the power of life and death in their fingertips, they didn't always. They weren't gods, or even demi-gods. In spite of all their skill, they fought the odds like everyone else. I sighed. Maybe it was no one's fault. It was the nature of the disease. My thoughts exhausted me as I tried to sort it all out in my head.

On the ride home, the quiet unnerved me. I glanced at my never-silent passenger now encased in her self-imposed personal cocoon. She'd gone somewhere in her mind where

I couldn't reach her. I reached over to touch her. "You want to talk?"

She didn't even look my way. She raised her left hand and let it fall leadenly onto her lap. I could see the tears glistening in her eyes, defying gravity. She moved her head from side to side saying no in a very un-Sharon manner.

Normally, Sharon did ninety-five percent of the talking when I drove, which suited me fine. She would pepper me with rhetorical questions. My closed-mouth approach to conversation behind the steering wheel could never hold up for very long. She was so dang persistent.

But not today. Not after this news.

I kept my eyes on the road but slowed down to below the speed limit. I began to caress her arm, leg, shoulder and neck, alternately. She seemed to soften and relax, somewhat enjoying her form of "silent treatment."

We came upon the Arkadelphia road sign on the

throughway. There, Sharon waved the palm of her hand up and down in front of her body. She stared straight ahead, as if by not making eye contact, she could find the strength to articulate her words. She focused on the windshield. "This is what I'm going to do…"

She delivered each sentence with slow deliberateness.

"I'm going to follow up with chemo when we return. I do not want pity. I want to keep my life as normal as possible. I want to stay at home if I don't get better." After a lengthy pause, she continued. "But for now I want to stop off and visit my son, Matt, in Illinois, for a couple of days. I also want to walk along the Natchez Trace on the way home. I've heard it's lovely."

"I think I can arrange that," I said lightly.

After that, something weird happened. I looked over at my wife and she looked at ease. Perfectly at ease. She had no tears or runny mascara, no red, puffy face, no smeared lipstick, no nervous gestures, nothing like what I expected to see from a woman who'd just been given a death sentence.

All I could think of at that moment was how serene she looked.

Odd as it sounded, I could *feel* Sharon's faith and determination in the car. It was as if she—and I, by virtue of breathing the same holy air as her—were wrapped in the spirit of Jesus.

I didn't say anything. If you picked my brain, you'd find I was still really pissed about the raw deal we'd gotten. Yet there I was, beginning to relax, little by little. I certainly had no desire to play our favorite song from the CD on the way back—it cut me to the heart to even think about what happened earlier and all that hope we'd harbored—but I wondered as I stole glances at my wife just how God's light got so deeply inside her...

I reached for her hand. When I can't find the words, somehow her touch always steadies me. I was so proud of her.

Chapter 14
A MATTER OF PERSPECTIVE

Though Sharon tried to continue teaching full time, the strain of handling more chemotherapy prevented her from having the strength to carry out her duties. She missed more and more days. Her dream had always been to see as much of the United States as she could. If she retired from teaching, she would be free to take longer excursions with me. I asked her to consider it. It didn't take long for her to decide.

"I've always wanted to see the Grand Canyon."

"So have I."

It was May 2006, not long after the trip to MD Anderson. We didn't need to have a great discussion or second-guess our decision to go west. She got on our trusty Dell computer and organized the first guided tour that we ever took.

She invited her son, Stuart, along and then arranged for the flights. Off we flew to Arizona. Our itinerary included a one-night stay in Phoenix where we took our rental car to see the sights. The solitary mountains that popped up in the urban sprawl interested her while an enormous billboard advertising homes to the tune of 2.5 million dollars boggled my mind. We drove around for about an hour trying to track down a home like that.

Stuart shook his head. "You guys, I'm telling you. We're not going to find one. They'll be in some kind of gated community."

Sharon made a face. "Aww, that's no fair. We can't see them from the road." She kept her eyes peeled for other natural scenery.

"Babe, those families might have an expensive home. But they don't have what we have."

"And what's that?"

"Each other." Very upbeat, I pointed to her and we simultaneously broke out singing our Sonny and Cher favorite, *I Got You, Babe.*

Stuart shook his head, clearly enjoying our spectacle. "You guys are a trip."

"Speaking of which, do you both remember how I almost tripped going down the aisle singing that song at our wedding?" *Ah, well, just another beautiful memory.*

"Hey, look at that enormous rock," Sharon exclaimed. "It looks exactly like an elephant—trunk, tusks, ears and all." She snapped photos as I drove by it. She had a fascination with rocks. I ought to know. Several that we found on our travels together now lay scattered in our front yard.

The next morning, we met with the tour director for Caravan Tours. We went over our itinerary, which included a number of natural parks, Sedona, the Grand Canyon and Las Vegas.

While we were in Sedona, we hired a female tour guide to take us on an off-road trip through the rocks and mountains. Thank God we had an excellent driver plowing through the rocky terrain. Sharon and I laughed later about not falling out of the jeep once.

Everything we saw turned out to be mystical and magical. Sedona exploded with color—russet, gold, several shade of brown, green and blue, with red rocks everywhere along with splashes of cloud-white across the sky. The area had a phenomenon called vortexes. We read that when a person stood in the midst of one, you could feel something happening to your hair and skin like the tingly sensations you feel when you touch a Van de Graaff generator. Some local people believed the Indian legend that the vortexes had healing abilities. Others attribute a long healthy life and vitality to vortexes

"If we could just find one, wouldn't that be great? If I stepped into it, I'm sure my cancer would be cured," Sharon said wistfully.

"I know." I tried to pin our tour guide down and locate one, but she said no one knew their exact location. You just came upon them by chance. We never found one. I guess it just wasn't our time.

"Oh! Look at that rock formation. It looks exactly like a crucifix with a cloud angel hovering over it. And the sky…Stuart, Joe, do you see that beautiful deep purple sky around it?"

"Mom, you and Joe are always talking about signs. Do you think that's a sign?" Stuart asked.

"Of course it is. What are the chances of seeing a rock that looks like a crucifix with a cloud angel hovering above? It's a sign all right, just like rainbows or butterflies appearing out of nowhere. It means that God is watching over us and hears our prayers." She squinted into her camera and clicked away. I was wondering if it would make her artist's canvas.

I clapped Stuart on the back. "Son, when a disease ravages you, you fight it with everything you have. You have to stay positive, and that means taking encouragement from Almighty God when He sends it. You don't want to miss His messages."

"Good point."

Sharon had stopped taking photos and seemed lost in thought.

"You ready?"

"Just thinking through what you said, Joe. Of course, our faith and optimism is based on our belief in God. Every good thing comes from him. But, but ... it's not just when people have serious things wrong with them, like cancer."

She paused and chose her words carefully. "That's where we get it wrong. We need to look to God with an air of expectancy every day, sick or healthy. It's not a 'desperation' kind of thing. Or not any more, anyway. God always wants to communicate with His children, through the Bible, or Godly counsel or whatever. We need to have an open heart to hear His voice in our circumstances, no matter what it is we're facing."

Stuart and I looked at each other, unsure how to respond. Finally, I said, "Agreed. What are you getting at?"

"Just thinking, that's all. I'm wondering, really, um, maybe I'm learning that it's not all about me getting well. It's about trusting God in whatever state I find myself in." She covered her mouth with one hand as her jaw dropped down. "Woooow, I didn't even know I was thinking that. Thank you, Jesus."

After sharing those thoughts with us, she seemed to

take in the sights with even more wonder and excitement, as if she'd suddenly released a burden she didn't even know that she was carrying.

The following day, we set out along with a full busload of other tourists to see the sights. The bus, decked out in floor to ceiling curved windows, had luxury upholstered seats with plenty of legroom for someone of my size.

As our bus headed north to Flagstaff on Interstate 17, we marveled how the red clay appeared to glow. The rock formations dazzled us. Sharon was in her element.

"Excuse me," she repeated as she moved from one side of the bus to the other snapping a dozen photos at a time. "Sorry," she'd say, crossing back again or leaning into another passenger to snap that special shot. No mere souvenirs of our trip, these would become fodder for the number of the land, sea and cloudscapes she'd paint.

As she focused the camera yet again, I saw a woman

who looked to be in her seventies smack her husband's legs. "Lean back, Burt. This sweet lady is trying to get a photograph of that clay rock formation." He obligingly twisted his body out of the way to allow her to get the shot.

"Thank you. I'm an artist, you know." She added modestly.

The elderly man's wizened face broke out in a wreath of smiles. "Doin' your research, huh?"

"Exactly."

The woman squeezed her husband's hand and said, "Aw, she's such a sweetheart, like our own daughter."

Stuart and I looked at each other. We didn't need to say how happy we were that the other members of the group took to Sharon so well. It was her show. We wanted to make it the best trip of her life. *That's what I say about all of them.* Funny, though. We never talked about any of the trips being our last. In fact, we always looked forward to what we'd see the next time we'd go to that place.

We exited the interstate and pulled up to the Grand Canyon Welcome Center. Although we sat in the middle of the bus, we straggled out, the last of twenty-odd passengers. As excited as Sharon was, she found it difficult to move quickly and keep up with eager group members.

"Ready to see it, Shar?"

"You bet."

We held hands as we went through the archway. I could feel her hesitate and then slow down as we approached the viewing platform. Her eyes grew wider the closer we go to the rim of the canyon. She let go of my hand and slowly raised her fingers to her face, covering her nose and mouth as tears welled up in her eyes. She then began to weep.

I expected to hear the "Hallelujah chorus," at that moment. Being the artist she was, perhaps she was caught up in the colors and all of their nuances. That's all I could guess. Without taking her eyes off the vista below, she reached back blindly, gripping for my hand to grasp and pulled it to her breast. She wanted me to feel her heart beating as we both became overwhelmed.

I didn't quite know how to respond.

"It's like watching you enter the Sistine Chapel," I whispered, in awe. I, myself, had never seen the Sistine Chapel but I'd heard people responded to it with the same extreme emotion.

She couldn't speak. Gulping for air, and sniffing, the tears continued to flow. I felt her heightened emotion in the rapid beating of her heart. Later, when we talked about the awe of this moment, we decided to call it "our Cathedral Moment."

Occasionally, Shar wanted to walk along the south rim of the canyon and take pictures. I limped along, trying to ignore the outcries of my screaming knees—a legacy of wear and tear from my college basketball days and my ill spent youth jumping out of trees. I also found myself wheezing. *As an athlete, you should have never started smoking. You're paying for it now, buddy.*

Sharon stopped to wait for me. "Are you okay, honey?"

"Never better."

That afternoon, we got something to eat in the little food court. I settled for two nicely packaged hotdogs. Grasping them in one hand, I picked up some ketchup, mustard and relish with the other. I needed a flat surface. Ah, a two-foot high stone wall near the edge of the canyon. *That'll do.* I set one of them down while I ripped open the condiments with my teeth and spread them on the buns, using the packet as my knife to spread the mustard and catsup. As I sank my teeth into the first hotdog, I noticed a squirrel perched on the wall eying what he thought was his dinner.

"I thought squirrels only ate nuts. I didn't realize they were hotdog connoisseurs."

Out of the corner of my eye, I spotted the squirrel approach the food. I was so angry that I wanted to give it a swat. But all I could do was try to slap it across its face as if to say, "How dare you!" like a woman in a Turner Movie Classic. Let me tell you, it's a lot harder to mess with a hungry squirrel's face than for those women to slap an uncouth villain. I made contact but had no idea if I hit its hard head, its chubby body or its furry tail.

Somehow when I did this, the hotdog and bun flew into the air. The momentum of my swing made me spin around and I watched the meat fly out of the bun. It landed on my back and slid down the backside of my shorts.

As I tried to stare down and shoo the offending squirrel

away, he just sat there in attack mode, snarling at me. I never thought a squirrel would behave like that. I figured all I needed to do was raise my hand and it would run away. That's how I scared other squirrels in my backyard. With this one and his friends, it was like a classic Mexican standoff. Somehow, and I still don't know how this happened, the hotdog landed back in the bun on the wall. I had a problem, though. Now it lay between the squirrel and me. As I reached for my food, the squirrel chittered angrily, as if to say, "Hey, big guy, go ahead and take my hotdog. Just see what happens."

By this time, the squirrels and I had attracted a huge crowd. I didn't know which one they were cheering for. I could feel the spectators' emotions swinging in favor of the squirrel. Someone said, "Mommy, why did that man smack the squirrel?" I heard another one say, "Leave that poor, defenseless squirrel alone."

How could I ever hope to convince them of what really happened?

Shar stared at me and gasped. "Honey, are you bleeding? I think the squirrel bit you on your behind." She lowered her voice. "What are those streaks? Oh. It looks like you uh, had an accident."

"Huh?"

She whispered. "I mean, like you pooped your pants."

I yelped and jumped backwards, feeling for puncture wounds and horrified that I could have soiled underclothing. "That damn squirrel!" My hand came back with traces of brown and red where my shorts had come into contact with the leaping hotdog and condiments.

Oh great! First I had to deal with this deranged squirrel, and then I had to deal a crowd of people thinking that some old man needs his adult diaper changed.

Shar took a whiff off my hand and laughed. "Ahhh, it's

only mustard and ketchup. Let me help you." She took some napkins, wet them with her bottle of water and dabbed at the stains.

As we were taking care of this, Sharon said, "Look honey, the squirrel is scampering over the wall with your hotdog. Isn't that cute?"

"Huh. Cute, my hungry, condiment-stained *ass*."

As we were returning home that evening, seasoned Grand Canyon sunset watchers kept reminding us to keep an eye on the rather bland looking sky. Amid all the comments to "wait," and "almost," someone called out to Sharon, "Mrs. Belan, get your camera ready…"

Suddenly, the western sky began to glow red, yellow and orange as we watched the colors spread north and south over the rim. I glanced at Sharon's face as she beamed and snapped pictures. The colors of the sky reflected in her eyes and on her face. I wish I had remembered to bring my camera. I wanted to capture her joyful expression forever.

A year passed. Sharon suffered through more chemotherapy treatments, in hopes of getting into remission. None of them worked for long.

One Saturday night we had several couples from church over to our house. Sharon was feeling well, and I prepared a lasagna dinner with an antipasto salad, garlic bread and iced tea. Sharon had outdone herself with a cherry pie for dessert.

The conversation turned to travel. "I've always wanted to go on a long cruise," one of the wives said. She challenged the group to a proposition. "What do you think about taking one?"

Sharon nodded. "What if we went to Alaska? I taught my second-graders about igloos, glaciers, Eskimos, and whale blubber, but I've never had the opportunity to learn first-hand about any of it. That would be cool."

I shook a finger at her. "In more ways than one."

My wife coughed. Her system always seemed to be run-down. But at least tonight she was headache-free and hadn't vomited in over two days. She'd just finished another round of chemo. We were waiting to see if that slowed down the cancer or not. She walked more slowly and tired rapidly these days.

"You hate the cold," I pointed out. "You're not teaching anymore either," I reminded gently.

"But this is different." She tossed her head. "It's an opportunity to see … I don't know… icebergs and whatever else Alaska has to offer its tourists." She looked determined.

Stan cleared his throat. "She's in remission, right? So, this is do-able, isn't it?"

She's never really in remission anymore.

I waited. Shar disliked it when people spoke about her, 'as if I'm not even in the room,' she'd said more than once. She knew they didn't do it on purpose but it still irked.

"Yes, *I* am." She braced herself to stand up to her full 5'5" height, sending a message that she was prepared to do what it took to get to Alaska now that it seemed in the works.

We scheduled the trip for June 2007.

For me, the trip didn't start out well at all. At the Erie airport, the TSA agent, a skinny little woman with a nasty expression on her face, glared at me. "Shoes off." I unlaced my sport shoes but apparently I didn't move fast enough to suit her because she said, "Step aside, sir," and made a motion for me to get out of the way. I looked around, wondering if anyone else had heard her speak to me with such impatience.

I took my time. At nearly seventy years of age, I was

no spring chicken. Add two surgically-repaired knees to that mix. I had no intention of speeding up just to please some TSA employee. I placed my shoes in a gray container and set it on the conveyor belt. *Shoes. Check. Two keys. Check. I don't have any change. Okay.* I moved ahead.

"Sir, it's not your turn." The agent motioned for me to stop. I did. Finally, he gestured for me to pass through. Wouldn't you know? The alarm sounded. I groaned. How could I forget to mention my double knee operation? I explained while he ran that damn wand over me. I looked around to see if anyone was annoyed with me for taking up all this time. That's when I saw Shar and the others waving from the other side of the metal detector. They'd gotten through with no difficulty.

I got the motion to go ahead. The alarm went off. Again. "What the—"

The agent told me to remove my belt, my watch and

asked if I had any coins in my pocket.

"I most certainly do not," I said. She motioned for me to check anyway. I reached into my pocket and found … a dime and a nickel. That earned me a thorough pat-down.

Then that rent-a-cop looked over her spectacles at me. *She must be thinking, yeah right, this guy can't be trusted.* So she took my carry-on bag and unzipped it. She dumped everything on the table and scrambled all the contents. "Sir, *these* are not permitted on board." She pointed to my fingernail clippers. What does he think I'm going to do with them? Brandish them at my fellow passengers and hijack the plane? I shook my head. Imagine having the kind of job where you are responsible for people's lives. Not one I'd enjoy. I wearily handed them over.

He tossed everything back in the bag and zipped it up. My underwear and socks lay tangled together. My medicines, meticulously placed in order of when I needed to take them, lay scattered in a heap to the side. I cursed. For the first time in my life, I wanted to strike a woman.

"Sir..." She motioned for me to take my shoes and move on. "You're holding up the line."

I fumed as I laced up my size 13 ½ triple E sport shoes, taking my time. Finally on the other side, I hissed to Sharon, "Did you see that?" I threw up my arms in mock-surrender. "Classic example of Murphy's Law." *I would have screamed once upon a time but nowadays, I could laugh at myself.* The only thing that really irked me was how she scrambled my belongings. "She would've received medals from the Third Reich." I said, half-seriously.

"Honey, think of the story you'll be able to tell," she said brightly.

"Yeah, I can tell everyone how I was abused by a woman."

The long delay in Erie forced us to speed to our

connecting flight after we arrived in Detroit. The group took off at a run. "Tell them to hold the plane, if you can," I shouted as I tried to snag a wheelchair for Sharon. *Got it.* I piled the carry-on bags in her lap. "Let's go."

Within minutes, the wheelchair pulled ahead. *Damn these knees.* "I'm coming," I called, limping behind as I panted and pumped my arms to reach them.

"Come on, Gimpy," Shar called back to me. I was going as fast as I could, and tiring rapidly. She, on the other hand, looked like she was enjoying every minute of the race. Her green eyes lit up as she held onto the bags. She was actually *laughing. It doesn't matter to her if we make it or not.* She won't be laughing if we miss the flight and our tour in Seattle, will she?

We finally reached the gate, only to find that it had changed to one on the other end of the concourse. Aghast, I stared at the others. "Don't tell me…" How would I ever get the energy to make it?

"What a blast!" Shar said, wiping what I could only guess were happy tears for the joyride she'd just taken across the airport. I shook my head in disbelief. "Let's try to make it." I had my doubts.

Again, we dashed madly across the concourse to the alternate gate. When we got there, we found the flight was delayed for an hour. Then the flight was canceled.

Shar pointed to the people all around the waiting room, "Look at everyone flipping their cell phones out to make new arrangements." She giggled. "This is so much like *life,* isn't it? We plan to the best of our ability how things will go, but life has a way of surprising us. It doesn't mean that it's *bad*—just different." She didn't seem to mind missing the tour in Seattle at all.

We waited in the long line to talk to the ticket agent and finally booked a direct flight from Detroit to Vancouver for the following morning.

"If only we'd left Erie on time," I groaned. "The airline doesn't care about us."

Shar smiled, trying to bolster our little group, "Look at how accommodating they're being. They're passing out vouchers for 25,000 free miles and food from the food court when it opens in the morning."

The rest of the group nodded, but they, too, seemed unhappy. A chorus of stomach growls sounded within the group. Hunger gnawed at everyone. "Look. The airport is going into shut-down mode. I wonder if the airlines are sensing a panic?" one of the men observed.

"They must be," his wife agreed. "The booking agents are leaving. Look at 'em. That whole group is taking off."

"I bet it's just the evening slow-down," Shar said, shrugging. "You guys, it'll be fun for us to stay here overnight because there wasn't enough time to travel into town, get lodging, and still be able to make it back to the airport in time to make our flight to Vancouver. Besides, we would have to go through security again before boarding our flight. We can sing and pray and maybe even sleep. Hey, I have a pack of peanut butter crackers. Anyone want one?"

"I wish I knew what happened to our luggage. Is it socked away somewhere here in the airport? Did it go on to Seattle or Vancouver?" I griped. I looked around. We had no one to ask.

Sharon and I cuddled on the floor. I kept her warm as best I could. She convinced me of how much fun the two of us would have. "It's an adventure. Another Excellent Sharon and Joe Adventure." She didn't seem put out at all.

"I think we can compromise and say it's a 'misadventure.' You're right. What's a trip, without a little spontaneity?" I grinned.   She put her head on my lap and I finger combed her hair, really the bangs of her wig. Her hair was just beginning to grow out. I looked over at her. Even in the dimmer light, I could see the tip of her mouth tilt up into a happy smile. I traced the outline of it with my finger and realized how she'd changed tonight's dismal outlook for me.

After several phone calls to the travel agency in Seattle, we learned we wouldn't get a refund for the missed one-day tour we'd scheduled.

"I understand it's not your fault," the agent said, "and you couldn't have canceled in advance. That's just our policy, I'm sorry."

"Well, it's a pretty stupid one," I grumbled under my breath as I ended the call.

"It's okay, Joe. We'll visit Seattle another time. We have the rest of our lives."

"Yeah, I guess it's not the end of the world." I was still

ticked, though.

In Vancouver, we went on to check about finding the shuttle bus. Easy enough to find but they had no record of our name on the shuttle bus list to the port to get on the ship. "So you're telling me you have no mention of Sharon and Joe Belan but you have the names of the rest of members of our group?" I was dumbfounded.

"We're obviously together," said one of the other guys. "Take our word for it. Besides, we are all wearing the same hats and T-shirts with the words Alaska 07."

I heard Shar say, "Let's see if we can find some food. Let our big strong husbands sort this out. They'll get Joe and me on that shuttle."

"Yeah, I'm so hungry. It's been a whole day since we've eaten."

My wife turned out to be right. We sorted out the problem in no time at all. They let us on the shuttle bus and we boarded our ship without a hitch.

An hour out of Vancouver port, everything changed.

"Look. The sun is poking through the clouds," my own little sunbeam reported. We stood on deck overlooking the waves. Little by little, the choppy seas calmed. The sun glinted off the water, making it sparkle.

"Amazing!" I whistled. "Up to this point, our trip to Alaska set the perfect stage for Murphy's Law, providing us with…what did you call them? *Perspective-altering opportunities*. I like that phrase. Now everything is smooth, beautiful sun, calm seas…"

"You know what it reminds me of? The clinical trial at MD Anderson. Going through all those hardships to regain my health. Remember the terrible flu symptoms? When the stem cells implanted, we thought we were headed for Easy Street." She laughed.

I frowned. *Why did she have to go and bring that up,*

right when things were starting to get good? "Let's not dwell on that time, honey, we're on an exciting adventure."

"That's my line." She smiled. "No, really. It reminds me of that time."

"But it didn't work." I looked out over the water. *And don't jinx this trip by comparing the two.*

"I don't know. Maybe it prolonged my life. Sweetheart, my point is, we were praying for the wrong thing. I wanted God to heal me. That was *my* plan, not God's. Once I stopped having my own agenda, I could see my life more clearly—and um, delight in it. Tomorrow isn't promised…"

This conversation was getting way too philosophical for me. "Sharon, let's just enjoy the trip," I pleaded.

She touched my back with her hand. "Joe, look at me. Something's been on my heart, and I really want to share it with you. It's important," she said, suddenly serious.

"What?" After a moment, I turned and gave her my attention.

"After all I—we've—gone through, I'm a little surprised it took so long for this truth to sink in on a gut level."

"What are you talking about, Babe?"

"Our day-to-day life is *the* journey. We don't get to choose how it goes. We can't control it, any more than you could control the way that officer went roughshod through your belongings in Erie, right? So we just need to enjoy the trip as much as what's waiting for us at our destination. We need both. It's all in our perspective."

I thought about it for a couple of minutes. Was she chastising me for how I responded to the difficulties of our trip? When I looked at her, I didn't see any blame. She just looked back at me with those earnest green eyes.

"That's easy to say...but when life throws itself at you

—"

"Honey, it's a matter of perspective. It's a choice."

I looked down at the water. She wasn't accusing me of anything but I wanted to defend myself. It was important to me that things went smoothly and as anticipated. "I don't take disruptions or changes of plan very well," I admitted.

"I haven't always either. I'm just saying, we shouldn't put ourselves in a pressure cooker. I think what God is teaching me through my cancer journey is to take it day-by-day and be grateful."

Suddenly, it was as if I'd heard a Hallelujah chorus. The light of her truth went off in my brain. I stared at Sharon. *How did you get so wise?* As big as I was, I felt small next to her. "You're absolutely right."

She looked over at me and grinned. "God is our instructor. And this cancer seminar sure is teaching us a lot. Life is our workshop."

"I guess we're all life-long learners," I observed. "And you said you had no interest in leadership training," I teased.

She slipped her soft arm around my waist and lay her head on my shoulder. "Thanks for this trip to Alaska, Joe."

"Thanks for sharing my journey, Shar."

The late afternoon sunshine made me sleepy. "Ahhh, this is the life," I said, stretching out my long limbs on a reclining lounge chair on one of the decks.

"Let's go for a walk and explore the cruise ship." Shar tugged on an arm.

I opened one eye. "Now?" I rubbed my knees. "Okay, up and at 'em." I removed my sunglasses. "Won't be needing these as we explore its innards, will I?" We set out hand-in-hand.

That day we started a routine of seeking out new areas on the ship every afternoon. I especially liked the galley.

My wife seemed to like nothing better than to meet new people and drink a cup of hot coffee on every ship excursion we took.

"Tomorrow we arrive in Anchorage. I can't imagine how landfall could be any better than the cruise we've just been on," I said, taking her in my arms and cuddling.

But it was.

The ship took us out mornings, afternoons or both on excursions. Oftentimes, we rode a smaller boat if our group wanted to see a specific island or attraction. Of course, the natural Alaskan landscape was stunning.

Typically on a tour, our guide pointed out, "Train your eyes on that glacier. Before long, you'll see a small section cave in and drop into the water. This is called *glacier calving*." Half an hour later, Shar was peering through her camera lens and grabbed my hand, "Look, Joe! That glacier is calving. Whoa! What a splash!" I turned just in time to see a section of ice crash into the water below. We were all shading our eyes and exclaiming by this time. "There are some blue ice floes," I said with equal excitement as a ton of blue ice came into view. Everyone wanted to know where, and then, suddenly, they saw it, too. Whole sections of ice reflected shades of blue until it almost looked purple.

"Why is it blue?" Jon asked our guide.

He responded with a very technical definition. I asked questions to learn more about it. Sharon summed it up rather simply. "So I guess it's blue because the ice is thinner in sections. And some red infra ray colors are absorbed...I just think it's pretty to look at it."

As we rounded one of the islands, the guide pointed out several eagle's nests high in the trees. "You are now looking at a protected species. By the way, just a fact you might like to know. The American Bald Eagle was removed from the Endangered Species list the day the ship set out from Vancouver harbor." We all clapped and whistled.

"We gotta protect our national bird," someone shouted.

Later that day, we encountered a gray mother whale swimming along with its calf. Again, Sharon caught it first. "Honey, what is that?" She pointed with her face and eyes.

I stared. "I don't know…I think it's a … is that a whale and its baby?" I asked the guide.

"It sure is." He grinned. "You folks are lucky. Not every tourist gets to see a mother whale and its calf."

Sharon caught her breath. "They're enchanting," she half-whispered. As she watched, I wasn't the least bit surprised to see tears rolling down her excited face. I had come to expect such reactions from her when something touched her.

Our cruise was winding down. We would arrive back at Vancouver the next day. As a final celebration, the cruise held a party with appetizers, open bar and a live band that provided dance music. Of course, we attended.

"Listen to this song…" Sharon held a finger up to draw my attention. "Do you remember a long time ago when we went on that Three Rivers cruise in Pittsburgh? The band played this song and we danced to it, I believe."

"How could I ever forget?" My voice sounded husky, even to my ears. As I looked over the water, I remembered that cruise as if it were yesterday. I even recalled the events leading up to it.

***

Pittsburgh, 1995

During the long-distance phase of our relationship, Sharon decided to visit me for the weekend. That Friday evening, she snuggled up to me on the sofa. "What part of

Pittsburgh will I see this weekend?"

"I thought we might go on a riverboat cruise. It takes us on the three main rivers here. How does that sound?"

As usual, she was game for any outing.

We drove into Pittsburgh from Monroeville, turning onto the Parkway heading west. "This is the same road you got lost on when you came to visit me for the first time," I pointed out. She gave me a don't-remind-me-about-that look. "What? I offered better directions than you could get from Yahoo. Oh there's the Penn Hills exit. Do you think I should take it?"

My teasing earned me a frown and I quickly changed my tune. "I was only kidding." I laughed nervously. Though we had been together for a couple of months, I still couldn't read her reactions that well. She would either laugh or feign displeasure, and the latter always threw me off, mostly because I tried so hard to please her.

She pretended to be displeased now. Or was she really mad? I gave her a furtive glance but heavy traffic forced me to keep my eyes on the road. She'd crossed her arms but had a fixed half-smile on her face. Had I gone too far? I went over the conversation again in my mind. I bit my lip. I hoped I hadn't offended her. Putting on my turn signal, I passed a semi. A couple minutes later, a driver threatened to cut me off and I lay on the horn. "Stupid driver," I mumbled.

Sharon shook her head. "Pittsburgh drivers. Never know about them." *What did that mean?*

After a short silence, Sharon started talking again. I looked over at her and smiled, relieved. We fell into a comfortable banter that lasted until we arrived at the wharf. I checked my watch. "We're here with almost an hour to spare."

"And I suppose you reserved this a month ago," she

teased.

"Just two weeks ago. I narrowly missed the cut-off number."

"In Erie, you can schedule things the same day or the day before. I'd never remember to reserve them in advance." She rolled her eyes. "Thank God, I have *you* for that."

We complemented each other that way. Everything in Pittsburgh needed to be planned ahead of time. It took me awhile to get used to the small-town feel of Erie and how quickly I could get reservations anywhere. Living in Erie made it easier to be spontaneous.

"Shall we board the river cruise?" I asked, extending my arm.

She took it, and we walked onto the boat. We hardly noticed the riverboat drift away from the wharf until we suddenly felt the thrum of the powerful engines as we headed upstream against the current of the Monongahela, or the "Mon," as people in the Burgh called it. If we continued in that direction, we would have eventually gotten to Morgantown, West 'By God' Virginia.

I wrapped my arms around Sharon. As she leaned into me, she pointed to the right. "What's that?"

"Hmmn? Where?"

"There."

I couldn't see where she was looking. I'd closed my eyes and was nuzzling her neck. She turned around and placed both arms around my neck before mouthing against mine, "the building with the big clock."

I knew it so well I didn't need to look. "The Duquesne Pilsner building," I murmured back, my eyes still closed. I kissed her fiercely then and even allowed my hands to wander. It didn't take her long to dispatch my roving hands back to her waist. She taught me her first lesson on propriety: no sexual touching in public. I actually liked that. An old-fashioned girl with social morals.

I pointed out the steel mill at Braddock and Kennywood Park up on the bluff in Duquesne. "The boat won't go that far, though." It swung around to head downstream on the Mon.

"Shar, they're calling us to eat. We sat down in our designated places. I continued. "We'll be able to see the early evening reflection on glass and steel buildings to our right. For a while, all you could hear was the clinking of silverware. We passed the Fountain on the Point, all lit-up. "That water for the fountain comes from the aquifer from below the bottom of the Ohio and Allegheny Rivers."

"I *love* geology. You name any rock and I'll tell you about it. I was the best in my college class." "Me too." Said Sharon.

"I bet you were. I guess that a boy from The Rocks,

McKees Rocks, that is, should know about rocks, too." I said with a smile.

She rolled her eyes at what she thought was my attempt at humor. Just then Three River Stadium caught her eye. She asked me about it.

"Would you like to catch a Pirates game there some time?" I asked, eager to offer myself as a guide.

She batted her eyes. "How could I turn down such a nice request for a date from a handsome stranger like yourself?"

"Ha. Is that your response to every handsome stranger that comes along?" She didn't answer me, the rat.

"You know so much about these three rivers. You're an expert on their history. Tell me the truth. You've worked as a tour guide, haven't you?"

"No, I just grew up here. I've seen these places all my life."

She smiled over at me. "I feel very lucky."

"There's Brunot's Island. Once upon a time, beautiful trees grew there. It had a park, a horse racing track, a marina and a beach on the northern end. Now it's just a dark, dirty slag heap where the Duquesne Light Company built it's power generating plant and dumps its waste cinders."

Sharon frowned at the water surrounding her. "I hate what industry does to our natural resources." She sniffed. With her hand, she fanned the air away from her at the railing and quickly covered her nose. "I see what you mean by the senseless dumping. It smells horrible!"

I covered my nose, too, and slipped into a very popular venting we locals fell into when it came to the sludge caused by these industries. "You should see the effects on the roads…each municipality buys the cinders which gets dumped on the icy roads in the winter." After a while, I realized we'd fallen into a negative mindset. In an effort to regain her smile, I launched into a new topic. "You see where the island juts out into the river? My mom and dad had some very romantic picnic dates there."

She playfully ducked behind me then, slipped an arm around me, and snuggled up against me. "I'm cooooollllddd. Umm, tell me some more about your parents' dates on the river."

"Let me warm you up first!" For a while I did just that, rubbing her arms and cuddling her in my arms. I never got back to talking about my parents.

The cruise continued down the river. At our backs stood the dark grey towers of Western Penitentiary, a maximum-security prison. I didn't want to ruin the moment by showing her the building that housed murderers and rapists. Instead, I pointed out my hometown of McKees Rocks. "The town's namesake rode his horse off the end of that mound called the Indian Mound, right into the river to escape the Indians who lived at the mouth of Chartiers Creek." I lowered my voice, "McKee was probably trying to 'make it' with the chief's daughter."

She thumped me on the back. "Joe..."

"No, I'm telling you the truth as I know it," I protested.

We passed under the bridge, which spanned the Ohio River from the "Rocks" to the North Side. "If we boys wanted to become men, as rite-of-passage, we had to walk across the bridge's superstructure from one end to the other. Most of my friends couldn't or wouldn't do it. It scared the hell out of me, but I did it. At that moment, I knew I was a man and could do anything I set my mind to doing. I was only sixteen years old back then." I laughed, remembering.

Sharon's mouth fell open. "Joe. No way! Really? So dangerous...and stupid!" She held me tighter. "Wow. Even the way you talk about this bridge ... I can see how these rivers make up, or maybe, contribute to who you and your family are today."

"Yeah, I guess so."

It might sound unmanly to say this but the rest of that evening felt magical. Maybe it was how we touched—how she leaned into me or how my hand felt so right on her back and around her waist—or it could have been the way the lights fell onto the water. Perhaps it was the music piped onto the deck or the dancing we did together. It could have been her signature perfume or a combination of all these and of course, the stories I shared.

During that one little boat ride, I handed my life to her on a platter. She saw in my eyes the love I had for my family and my hometown. She heard in my voice the pride I had in the history of my beloved three rivers. She could smell along with me the air of the dying river town industries. On this night I knew that once I opened my heart to her, I could never close it. Ever.

***

"You know, Shar, it was still early days in our relationship when we took that cruise. We'd been dating, a couple of months? I didn't know when you were teasing me and when you weren't back then."

She smiled. "You still don't sometimes."

"What I've learned since then, though…that a look, a tilt of your head, it all says something special about you … and us."

"Aww, Joe. That's so sweet."

"We knew from the beginning that we were right for each other, didn't we?"

"Yes. What a beautiful memory. I'm glad we took that

cruise. Even though we hadn't voiced our feelings yet, our love just *flowed* like the river that night, and it's never stopped," Sharon said softly.

I couldn't resist playing on her words. "You mean like the *blue ice floes*? Except *our* ice is not thin," I hastily added. *Incredible. After bad relationships, we both got new chances at love...and intimacy.* "My knees might not be up to what they were way back then, but they still work. Shall we?" I stood up and led her out onto the dance floor.

"How can I turn down a request from such a handsome stranger as yourself?" she asked with a grin.

Chapter 15
SHARON'S BIG NIGHT

"I'd like to celebrate my birthday this year with a party," Sharon announced, pen in hand. She looked up from where she sat at the dining room table.

Oh my God. A long silence hung in the air. *What do I say? "Honey, you look a wreck." Out of the question. I can't ask her if she's sure she's up to it. She'll think I'm being over-protective-- again.*

"Do you think more will come right on my birthday or that Friday night?"

Will people come? If they do, will they treat the party like a wake? Will they stare and act morose? Or will they look away?

I can't say, "It's probably not a good idea. We have no idea how you'll be feeling the day of the party."

She'll just stare, fold her arms and look away. I'll feel terrible.

I have to get this just right. How do I answer?

It's just a party for God's sake, nothing else. We've had all kinds of parties since we've been together. This is not the bomb you think it is. But I'm used to seeing her this way. Other people aren't. Will they feel uncomfortable?

Just say "Yes, that's a great idea, hon." You know that's what she expects you to say.

Shar leaned over in my direction. "What do you think? The house is too small for the number of people I'd like to invite. I think we'll have to have it somewhere else."

She has no idea that I even doubt this party should take place.

"Well honey, how many were you thinking of having?"

"Forty or so."

I thought for a few minutes. "Well…"

"Joe, remember that little German club …
Siebenbuerger's? I used to take you there when you came
to visit me. Do you know the one I mean?"

I jotted the name down. "Yeah. It's just a few miles
away from our place, right? Sounds like a good place. Shall
I call and see if it's free on that date?"

"Perfect. Now, help me with the names, honey. You're
the list-maker. Write them down. I don't want to forget
anyone."

*I guess I'm in now. No trying to convince her
otherwise, And why should I? If she wants a party, then I'll
make sure she gets the best one ever.*

I helped her make up the guest list—family, friends,
church members and former teaching colleagues. Some of
the people on the list hadn't seen her for quite a while,
before the Alaska trip, a good two years ago. A lot had
changed since then, health-wise.

Before we sent out any invitations, we had to get a fixed location. I found the number to Siebenbuerger and punched it into my cell phone. "Yes, yes... more than a month away. The evening of March 26. More like six o'clock. Yes, I'll wait while you check...no kidding? It's *free? Beautiful.*" I turned to Sharon. "It's..."

"I heard. *Great.*" Sharon's face looked flushed. She looked ready to hunker down and do some work. "I was thinking we could send some invitations by email, and the rest through the post office," she said, sensibly.

"You do the email invites. I don't like computers. Rather, they don't like me." I made a face.

"Okay, deal. Joe, we need to make sure to add a line about "No presents." This is just a get-together that happens to be on my birthday. Would you mind helping address the envelopes of the ones we send out?"

"I think I can do that much," I teased, "and if your sons

will be so generous with their time, they can help me decorate the place."

"Oh, I'm *sure* they'll help. They'll do anything for their mom." Her green eyes sparkled, lighting up her drawn face. "And we'll have to have music, so that means a DJ. What about Paul? He's a professional. If I asked him, I bet he'd bring all of his Oldies music for us to dance to. I'm going to call him right now." She bubbled over with excitement.

"Joe!" She grabbed my hand. "I know one song we *have* to sing. Louis Armstrong's *What a Wonderful World.* I *looove* that song." She began humming it. She stopped and absently tapped the pencil as she thought out loud. "Oh dear. Not everyone will know the words. I need to type them out so we all have a copy. Yes, I'll *do* that." She scribbled a note to herself.

I dropped a kiss on her neck. I loved watching Sharon

in action. She didn't usually have a plan and a purpose for everything she did. But this time she did.

I hadn't seen her so excited for a long time. This party gave her something to focus on and pour her energies into —what little she had, anyway. She lingered over the daily mail, opening all the RSVPs without delay. She checked her email often. A few days before the party, she walked into the kitchen where I was preparing our dinner and put her arm around my waist. "Guess what? Oh, Honey, guess what!"

"What?" I asked, loving her familiar touch.

"Every one of the people we invited has accepted. This is my last RSVP," she crowed, waving an envelope. "One hundred percent! How does that happen in this day and age?" She hugged herself in excitement.

"Wow."

"I know. I can't *believe* it." She did a little tap dance

and I couldn't resist taking her in my arms and doing a slow turn and dip with her.

"This is going to be *some* party, Babe."

"Oh it *is*. Everyone is coming. Yaaay*!* I can hardly believe it."

"I don't doubt it. You'll be the 'Belle of the Ball'." I took her in my arms and kissed the peach fuzz she had for hair. "It's starting to grow out," I observed, my lips close to her skin.

"I know. I'm so happy." She gave me a rueful look. "But not fast enough for the party." She bit her bottom lip. "It doesn't matter, does it?"

"Not at all. You have some really great wigs. We can choose one together if you like."

"You're right." She pressed her face to my chest and closed her eyes for a moment. They popped right open again. "I went shopping with my sister and bought a beautiful outfit for the party. Shall I model it for you now?"

"How about we wait and you surprise me? I might not be able to control myself today." I gave her the once over and lifted my eyebrows suggestively. The truth was, she looked tired.

The night before the big event, she lay curled up into me. "I'm so excited. I can't wait for the party tomorrow. What a gift from God." She released a deep, contented sigh. Before long, I heard regular breathing and knew she'd fallen asleep.

I didn't want anything to go wrong and disappoint her. *Lord, let it be a happy occasion and let her strength hold out.*

Toward the end of the next afternoon, we men in the family surveyed our work. The streamers hung in place. Scores of colored hand-blown balloons hung from the ceiling in balloon bouquets. The tables sported white paper coverings laced with confetti and each one contained a filled candy dish in the center. Finally, Stuart finished hanging the big Happy Birthday sign.

"Good job on the banner," I said. "You found the grommets. Each letter swivels in a different direction. It looks perfect."

Stuart smiled. "Glad to do it. Like my mom said, we'd do anything for her. Right, Matt?"

Matt nodded. He had a bunch of napkins in hand and was placing some at each table. "You got it, bro."

"I heard that," Shar called, "and love you guys." She clasped her hands to her breast and then blew a kiss to each of the men in her life, including my son, Jason.

The DJ quickly set up and began playing music when the guests arrived.

Sharon stood in the middle of the room. Someone thrust a festively-wrapped gift with curly blue ribbons into her hand. "Oh, you didn't need to give me a gift. Your presence is gift enough," she admonished. "So *glad* you could come, Frances. And this is…?"

"My husband, Jerry," Fran murmured.

"So nice to meet you, Jerry." Shar offered up her cheek and he kissed it.

She turned and saw another old friend. "Paula, I can't believe it. You look *wonderful*. Are you still doing the Leadership Workshop at Gettysburg each year?"

"I have been, but I'm getting ready to retire next year so that means no more workshops. This is a little something for you," she added, handing Shar a long rectangular glittery box with a big red bow as she hugged her.

"Paula. Thank you. I wish you hadn't."

I saw Shar point in my direction. "Joe's over there. He'll want to talk to you right away—probably shop talk. But don't you let him." She grinned.

The guests all took an interest in Sharon's health.

"How are you feeling?" they'd ask.

"I have good and bad days," she responded honestly. "Today's one of my better days."

When I looked up next, Shar had a huge crowd around her. She'd never moved from the center of the room. Surrounded by people she loved, I could hear her laughing and crying, asking about their lives and offering up memories of their shared time together. Her cheeks were flushed—but in a good way. She glowed. It made me think of our wedding day. She'd been a bubble magnet then—all the bubbles had circumvented me and gravitated to her, just like the crowd pressing in on her today. I told Paula as much.

She laughed. "Tonight I'd say she's more like a rock star. Everyone wants a piece of her. Look. They're holding out cards to her." She poked me in the side. "Joe, that guy's waving his pen. It looks like he wants her autograph."

Paula sounded very amused. "Darn. Didn't think of asking for one." She laughed.

I chuckled. "That's Mark. He does everything at the last minute He must have just signed the card and thrust it in her hand after he arrived. Good ol' Mark."

In a short lull that followed, I heard Shar say, "No, no getting out of it. I want to see you dance tonight. Back in the day, you were quite the dancer…" Sharon remembered something special about everyone. She welcomed each one of them into her midst as if they alone were the reason for the party.

I have to admit that I got a kick out of watching her get all this attention. She loved these people. They loved on her right back. No one seemed shaken or sad to see how Sharon had changed. Our eyes met for an instant as she hugged her aunt. She held up the many unexpected birthday cards in one hand, her jaw slack with surprise. The sparkle was back in her eyes, big time.

The waiters and waitresses filed into the room ready to take the orders.

I announced, "Ladies and gentlemen, please take a seat. Decide what you want to eat and drink because it's time to fill our bellies now. We have all evening for this love-fest."

As we waited for the food and drinks to arrive, several camera flashes popped up around the room. Shar's brother-in-law said, "Hang on. I need to capture the spirit of this night. Sharon. Smile," he called. She'd done nothing *but* smile since the first person arrived. *All anyone needs to do is focus a video camera on Sharon's face.* She was transparent in her joy.

After we finished eating, Sharon stood up, cupped her hands around her mouth like a megaphone. Before she spoke, a teacher friend sprinted up to the table. "Sorry to interrupt but I didn't want this gift to get lost." She handed Shar an oblong jeweler's type box with floral wrapping and a pale violet bow before ducking away. A ripple of laughter echoed around the room.

"You guys are the *best*. Really special. I told you, though, *no* presents. This party is my gift. You…you are my gifts, this year. Do you know what your friendship means to me?" Her voice cracked. The room grew silent and I heard some people sniffle around me. I elbowed a friend. "I think she's feeling a little overwh—" I choked, unable to get the words out.

I pointed to Jason and Stuart. They discreetly left the room and came back holding a white sheet cake decorated with red roses. In beautiful lettering across the cake, it read:

Happy Birthday, Rose of Sharon.

"Let me explain the inscription on your cake, honey."

It combined her love for roses, the Bible, and, of course, her name, which I'd been playing on. The biblical definition of *sharon* literally referred to a coastal plain in Israel. The rose of Sharon could mean a lily or a hibiscus or even a crocus, but for sure indicated a beautiful flower in the midst of other plainer flowers. "Shar, you might not be an actual rose but you are this flower."

"Oh, sweetheart—I don't deserve it."

"You do, and even more. It's in the Song of Solomon. In the next verse, he's telling his lover how much he values her. Do you know what he says?"

She shook her head, mystified.

"'*Like a lily among thorns is my darling among the maidens.*' This is exactly the way I feel about you after fourteen years of being together."

"Awww. You're so romantic." She leaned over and slowly kissed me.

It was as if everyone in the room disappeared and we shared that moment, just the two of us, until we heard whistles and catcalls and some clapping. Someone said, "Why don't you ever say things like that to me?" I turned to Sharon. "I'm fortunate. No thorns on this rose."

Sharon patted my face. She looked at the cake. Two large candles—a six and a two—sat in the center. Jason lit them. "Make a wish, mom," Stuart called. "Then blow out your candles."

The crowded room filled with laughter. Shouts of "Go ahead." and "one-two-three blow!" followed.

"I have to say this is the most wonderful birthday I've ever had," Shar said as she looked out at her family and friends and clasped my hand to her side.

"You say that every year." I placed a hand on her shoulder and gently massaged it. *Next year will even be better.*

She closed her eyes for a good thirty seconds, seeming to take the wish part to heart, and took a couple of deep breaths, leaned over and blew. For a moment, only candle smoke hung over the table. Then, the candles re-lit themselves.

"I should've known. *Trick* candles." Everyone laughed, and cheered her on. "Okay, here I go agaaaiiinnn."

Watching the candles relight themselves reminded me of how resilient Sharon herself was. We'd been fighting her cancer now for nearly seven years. She'd been down but always resurfaced … with new light.

As she blew them out, I scrambled to the utility kitchen, found a small Styrofoam bowl and filled it with water. She'd need it to douse the candles. After all, she couldn't keep blowing them out indefinitely.

As I returned to the cheerful group and Sharon, I thought about how early on I'd been worried about having the party. She was holding up fine. Her idea to have this party had turned out exceptionally well.

I picked the six up before it re-lit and as soon as she blew out the two, I dropped both candles into the shallow bowl of water. At the completed ritual, everyone clapped and cheered.

Sharon went about cutting the cake, while I passed it out. Finally, she sat back down and focused on her own cake. "It looks so smooth and lovely that I hate to wreck the design just to *eat* it. She touched it with her fingertip. "It's feels like satin," she said in a hushed voice. She tasted the tiny dollop on her finger. "Mmmm, creamy." she said.

"Come on, hon. Take a bite."

She picked up her fork and cut into it and popped it into her mouth. "Ohhhh. It's *heavenly.* Just as I thought… some kind of *rose* flavoring in the frosting." She licked her lips and cleaned the frosting off the fork. "Aside from the frosting, the cake is buttery and very moist." She ate the entire piece, which I made sure was a corner portion, knowing her sweet tooth.

After Sharon took her last bite, she blotted her lips with a napkin and stood up. "I'd like to ask you to do something to make this event even *more* special. Humor me, please. If we could all stand up, form a circle and hold hands, I'd like for us to sing Louis Armstrong's rendition of *What a Wonderful World.* I have copies for those of you who don't know the song or can't remember the words." She distributed small handouts to each person.

I could see elements of Sharon's teaching come through as she quickly organized the group. With the lyrics in hand, I predicted even the reticent singers would participate.

"The optimism and the colors of this beautiful song touch my artist's heart, and I hope the words touch yours, too, as we sing it together," she said. Then my lovely Sharon, who couldn't carry a tune in a bucket, spoke the words to the song ahead of the music.

As she spoke of how the roses bloomed, she looked at me and clasped my hand. *Yes, the roses had bloomed for both of us.* She pointed to several people around the room and mouthed the words, "For you. For you. For you." before she finished the stanza.

I misted up singing of bright blue skies and white clouds. The way she made me view clouds these days…I'd never be the same. I actually *saw* bears and bunnies—yes, me, the objective male science teacher—saw *bunnies*, and all kinds of creatures when I looked at the sky now. Sometimes I even pointed them out to her.

Oh, God, how she'd *changed* my life.

I squeezed her hand as my throat clogged with the next words. How could I ever doubt that I lived in a wonderful world when I had only to look at Sharon to remind me of my blessings?

Sharon read out the next few lines—how pretty the colors of the rainbow in the sky looked—as the group sang after her. Tears trickled down her face. The guests stole glances at her, and a few dabbed at their own eyes. I took out a handkerchief and blew my nose.

The next words focused on the beauty of friendships. With a single gesture, she seemed to shake hands with each guest en masse. Sharon voice broke as she read out, "how…d'you…do?" and she touched her heart and whispered, "I love you" through her tears.

When she got to the part about babies and watching them grow, she laughed, tears coursing down her face, and shrugged. "Babies do cry. What can we do?" I couldn't imagine a teacher more dedicated to her "children." It was always her goal to awaken their curiosity and get them excited about the world. I wanted to tell her again how much I loved that about her.

As we finished singing, I realized that our circumstances might not be exactly what we want, but we really do live in a wonderful world. Jason poked fun at me, pretending to rub his eyes with his two fists. I guess he got a kick out of seeing his old man with streaks of tears coming down. I must have looked goofy. But it didn't matter. I heard an awful lot of nose-blowing going on, and glances at other men told me even they had tears welling in their eyes. I did glimpse a couple of people who looked embarrassed by the public display of emotion. I think the older you get, the less you care. Shar had touched everyone with her life.

I gave an it's-out-of-my-hands gesture. "Don't give your dad a hard time."

With the food behind us, Paul started up the music and

the real fun began. Shar went around encouraging reluctant dancers. "Come on, just one, that's all I'm asking. Look at your wife (or husband). The dance floor is waiting for you both…" she'd say in an engaging voice.

One look at my wife and it was clear that she was having the time of her life. Though her face was wet from perspiration and swollen from the chemo, we saw that beautiful smile and the sparkling green eyes that reflected the life she still had.

Her shoulder-length brown wig wouldn't stay properly in place on her head as she danced. She didn't seem to care, and no one seemed to notice. I couldn't believe how effortlessly she still moved. My knees were killing me, but I couldn't decline a single time. This evening was turning out to be one to remember. The song was a fast one and I had to lead. It's as if my feet and arms remembered all by themselves. We still danced together perfectly, as if we were molded for each other.

A slow dance came and I welcomed the chance to hold my charming wife again in my arms and twirl ever-so-slowly. Who would've ever guessed that that first dance would lead to the beautiful slow dance our *life* had actually become. I ached for this moment to last.

At the end of the party, people pitched in to clean up, put away the chairs and sweep the floor. They kept hugging Sharon and talking to her as she stood on the sidelines. Her shoulders slumped, and she took a long breath. But the smile never left her face.

As I slid her Happy Birthday banner into a bag, I said, "What a superb night, Shar."

She nodded. "No one wants to leave…"

"…you. Nobody wants to leave *you*. They're even willing to clean up to stay around longer." I added putting my arms around her. "You made this party beautiful by weaving your special magic on everyone."

"Oh, get out of here. I did not."

I shrugged, as if to say, *you can try, but there's no denying it.*

To our surprise, someone cued the D.J. who we thought had already packed up. He played Louis Armstrong's song again just for Shar and me. "Go ahead, dance this last one," urged those who hadn't yet gone. "We'll wait this one out." With our arms tightly grasping each other we managed to rock back and forth to the rhythm of the music as we cried again.

"Thanks, Paul, for that song and all the other wonderful songs you put on for us tonight," Sharon said, giving him a hug and quick peck on the cheek.

I paid the bill, loaded up the car with the help of Sharon's sons and headed home. Sharon scooted across the seat to cuddle up next to me. She hugged my arm and put her head on my shoulder. It felt so good that I drove extra slowly all the way home.

What a big night for my wife, for us. As I slid into bed, I leaned over to tell her that I loved her. I whispered so close that she could feel my breath on her neck. I wondered if it tickled her. "We'll have an even bigger party for you next year," I said.

"Mmm," she murmured, her eyelids heavy, closing. She didn't say anything. I wanted her to say she couldn't wait for that one either. Somehow I needed for her to say it. But why?

How ridiculous. Of course she'd be around. I still had a lot of roses to buy her. She had a lot of clouds and rainbows yet to point out to me. *We'll still be skipping off into the sunset when I'm eighty and she's seventy-four. Well, with my knees, maybe I won't be skipping. Probably more like we'll be staring off at some unusual cloud shape instead with the smell of apples in the air.*

I held onto her that night with a kind of defiance, a fierceness that made my heart ache with something that I didn't want to identify. Long after she fell asleep, I lay awake, my eyes dry but hot as I held the tears back. How could I feel this way after such a perfect evening, after such a perfect marriage?

In the dead of night the lyrics to Louis Armstrong's song only made me feel worse.

Chapter 16
CARING FOR SHARON

I stared at Sharon, shocked at how her condition had changed overnight. Hot to the touch, the severe edema made all her skin shiny and tight. She looked miserable. "Where do you hurt?"

"Headache. Pressure here." She touched her chest and abdomen. "My fingers … toes … tingling. I guess I'm having another bad day." She sighed.

Her voice sounded tight, as if it hurt her to move her mouth.

If you want to call your entire body filling with fluids to the point there is not one single wrinkle on your body a bad day, then yes, you're having one. But I'd call it more of a medical emergency.

I tried to keep the panic out of my voice. "Honey, let's

get you to the hospital."

In urgent whispers, I spoke to Dr. Sturm, "…need to have someone look at her immediately…not good…bring her right in then? … go through the ER? I'm out of here."

I sounded terse but we didn't have a moment to lose. Could this be life-threatening? My gut said it was. With my heart beating erratically, I closed my eyes to calm down and think clearly. *Should I have called an ambulance? No, that would've only scared Sharon. Get a move on, Joe.*

"Shar, honey, we need to get you to the hospital."

She struggled to open her eyes. They fluttered for a few seconds then closed again. She didn't make a second attempt.

"I'm going to put you in the back seat of the car, okay? I'm sure you'll be fine soon. We just need to do something about the swelling and your pain."

I knew my voice *sounded* calm but the feeling eluded

me.

She raised an arm as if she knew she'd have to be carried. I carefully placed it around my neck and gently scooped her up. I laid her on a soft cotton blanket, intending to wrap her with it in case she felt cold in the air-conditioned hospital.

"I'm right here," I assured Sharon from the front seat. "I'm driving safely, don't worry."

We checked in at the ER, and the doctor on duty took Sharon at once. Afterward, he spoke with me. "Mr. Belan, let me explain our current situation in regard to your wife's care. Unfortunately, we will have to wait for a room to become available. When one is ready, we'll get Mrs. Belan checked in and situated. Until that time, she will remain in the emergency room. A nurse will continue to monitor her vital signs to ensure her safety."

"Is she going to be all right? What's causing this?"

The doctor stared down at his clipboard, avoiding my gaze. "I'm sorry, Mr. Belan. I haven't received the necessary records to assess her situation yet. When I liaise with her other doctors, I'll have a better idea of what's causing it. Our current plan of action is to filter the excess water out of her system."

"Can I see her?"

"At the moment, a better way for you to help her is to fill out a separate admissions form so that when a room frees up, she can move right into it. Will you do that for her? You can see her after that. Take a deep breath. I can see you're stressed. Don't worry, she's in good hands." He rested an arm on my shoulder for a moment.

I could hardly think to fill out the paperwork. Date: What was today's date? I looked around for a calendar. July what … what … seventeenth? 2009. Patient Name: Sharon Belan.

After I finished the paperwork, the nurse took me to sit with my wife. She and I waited several more hours. But by early afternoon, she had a room.

Once we got into the room, things went more smoothly. Sharon was resting and I was working on a crossword puzzle.

"Fifty-three across: *Chopin piece.* Five letters long." I paused and mumbled to myself, "How about some help here? Forty-three down: *power failure.* That's easy—OUTAGE. So Chopin's piece begins with an 'e.' Hmmm." As I sought out another clue, I heard a light rap on the door. It slid open and a gentleman in a white hospital coat stepped in the room.

I pushed my puzzle aside.

"Mr. Belan? I'm Dr. Jon Cartright. How are you doing?"

"As well as expected."

He gave a rueful smile. "Right. Never good at this stage of the game. My position here is known as a Palliative Care Physician. It's just a fancy name for a doctor in charge of counseling families and patients in medical crisis. I'm heading up Sharon's team and will be coordinating her treatment from here on out."

"Of course, she's the star of the show," I joked. Apparently Shar's condition had gone way beyond our regular physician's capabilities. "Should I wake her?"

He glanced at my wife. "No, in her condition, it's best that she rest. We need to monitor her and do some tests beforehand. The edema, which is the swelling you see, can become toxic. So our priority is to remove the excess water from her system. We will eliminate it through a special dual-dialysis-like procedure."

"How does that work?"

"It's not a regular dialysis, per se, but it works in a

similar manner. As we drain the excess water out of her system, we'll be putting the electrolytes, corpuscles, the white blood cells, all the parts of the blood she needs back in," he explained.

"When will we start that?" I asked, hoping it would be immediate.

"We're monitoring her for the time being. It'll probably be tomorrow or the day after. It's a slow process, so be prepared for that.

I thought of the stem cell process and sighed. I wondered how the two procedures compared.

The doctor said he'd be back in the morning and a nurse would be by soon to take some more vitals. "Anything you need, any concern you have, let me know. I am Sharon's advocate. This, of course, extends to you."

"Thank you." As wee shook hands he handed me his card and I turned back to my puzzle. Thirteen Down: A

Frock…

The dialysis began the next day, and went on for about forty-eight hours. They'd already taken eight liters of water out of her and were still going strong. Nervously joking I said, "Don't forget to put the other stuff back in. She needs all she can get."

"We'll do our best, Joe."

Sharon touched my arm. "What time is it? Honey, you need to go home. Take a shower."

"Try to save your voice," I begged, dropping my own down a decibel. "I'm perfectly fine here. Do I smell that bad?" I turned away from Sharon to check my armpits. *Ugh. I really need a shower.* I didn't feel comfortable leaving her. Though not normally paranoid, it seemed odd to me that the nurses were more preoccupied with the in-room computers than responding to the actual patients. I started to believe that they were playing video games. It was becoming a pet peeve of mine.

Time for a shift change. The incoming nurse checked on Sharon. She was fiddling with the damn computer. Of course, she didn't even glance Sharon's way. I gave an exaggerated sigh. "Why do you conduct your business that way?"

"Excuse me?" she said, still preoccupied with the computer.

I shook my head. "As far as I know, nursing is still a people-oriented profession."

The nurse gave me a blank look and smiled nervously. "Everything is as it should be, Mr. Belan." She took Sharon's pulse, then expertly cuffed her arm and pumped up the small rubber apparatus. She looked at the dial of her instrument. Satisfied, she annotated the pressure reading. "You doing okay, dear?" she asked.

She'd do a lot better if you'd get away from that stupid

computer first.

A day later, my pet peeve turned into a legitimate scare. Sharon began to retch. Right in the middle of that, she had a coughing attack and couldn't catch her breath. Of course, I pressed the call button immediately, and the nurse came running.

But instead of attending to Sharon, she went directly to the computer, turned it on and searched through several menus.

I couldn't believe my eyes. My wife was *choking*. "What are you doing?" She ignored both my wife and me while she continued to peck out hidden instructions on the computer. I lost my cool and got in her face. "Do something to save my wife from choking to death on her vomit!"

"Sir, our primary protocol is to make sure that Sharon's medications are not causing her choking."

Does that make sense? By all means seek out that information but let the poor woman choke to death in the process. We didn't go through the hell we did for seven years in trying to save Sharon's life only to lose it because a damn stubborn nurse wouldn't stop my wife from gagging on her own throw-up as she tried to catch her breath.

No way lady. I said through clenched teeth, "You need to attend to my wife."

The nurse abandoned the computer and went to Sharon, turned her on her side and cleaned the vomit from her mouth. At last, Sharon stopped choking. My wife had a terrified look in her eyes as tears rolled down her red face. She clutched onto my arm as best she could. She didn't have much strength.

My pulse raced at even the thought of what could have just happened. I saw red spots in the air and had to turn away to calm myself down. I bent over and held my wife in my arms, rubbing her back until I felt the tension leave her. She breathed more normally now that her coughing fit had ended.

As I stood up again, my head reeled. *What was that nurse thinking?* I'd worked as both a coach and a physical education teacher for several years. I was trained to deal with any physical problem, first. Then deal with the secondary issues. First Aid 101.

I would have attended to her myself but didn't want to interfere with hospital regulations. But by God, if that nurse had kept stalling, I would've had to jump in and save her. What else could I have done?

"I'll be right back, darling. "I'm going to pick up a newspaper. Do you want anything?" I asked, trying to hide the fact I needed to get out and let off some steam. *Sharon has been through enough without having to deal with my issues.*

She shook her head.

I'm trying to be calm, sweetheart. I am. But I am not ready to lose you like this.

Dr. Cartright wasn't in his office. *Great.* So much for Sharon having an advocate.

I headed outdoors. The July heat seemed stifling. I paced for a while outside the hospital. Then I took off down State Street, almost racing. My thoughts jumbled in my head. I couldn't live without Sharon. I needed her. We had been inseparable for nearly fourteen years. *God Almighty, help me. I'm not ready to give her up. Give me more time with her. I'll become patient. She's the reason I get up every morning. Don't take her away.*

There I was, still bargaining with God seven years after the diagnosis. I couldn't accept it. Just couldn't. Today's brush brought me face to face with her mortality.

I didn't know the tears were even coming down my

face until they trickled onto my neck. I brushed them away, angrily. I could feel panic setting in. *I'm not ready for this crossroads!* I still wasn't ready to give her up. I couldn't turn her over to God yet. I *wanted* her. In whatever form God chose to give her to me—no, *not* whatever form. I offered God a simple checklist. Sick. Healthy. You choose, God, but don't take her.

I wanted to scream. But I held it inside. As I wove in and out of the people along the State Street—shoppers, teenagers carrying boom boxes and mothers with small children, I heard one lady say, "If you don't speed it up, I'm gonna switch your hide good."

I winced. *Poor kid.* I concentrated on the sound my feet made when they hit the sidewalk. Finally, exhaustion took over and I returned to the hospital.

Inside the room, Sharon's eyes riveted to mine. She reached out to me. "Are you okay?"

"I'm fine." I faked a smile. "Newspaper?" *See. Just doing an errand.* "Want me to read it to you?"

"No news is good news." She pointed to a book on her tray. "I'd like you to read me something from this book."

She handed me Erma Bombeck's *A Marriage Made in Heaven or Too Tired to Have an Affair.* It was the perfect selection. We laughed all the way through the chapter. It felt really good to let go. I was guessing by Shar's laughter and a glimpse of her old smile, she felt the same way.

Dr. Cartright was back by the first of August, and we sat in Sharon's room, discussing her situation. His eyebrows furrowed, and he didn't smile. I took Sharon's hand in mine. "This is the part of a doctor's job no one ever likes. But it needs to be said. I'm sure you already know that things are not looking very good for you. Some people in this situation have not recovered. Some have. We can keep you in the hospital here but many people prefer being in their own surroundings. There's really nothing else we can do here but keep you comfortable and medicated to ease your pain. You can do that at home with Hospice—"

"We don't need Hospice," I said firmly. "I've worked around sick people for quite some time. I will care for my wife."

"Okay, you discuss it between the two of you. If you decide you'll be happier for Sharon to move back home, we have a checklist of equipment and supplies you'll need to get. Great Lakes Hospice will deliver them right to your home and set them up. If you prefer to care for your wife, that's fine. They offer a number of supplemental services that make a difference in homecare. The number for Hospice is at the bottom of the paper. Give them a call for the hospital equipment, and keep the number in the event that you need them to do anything. We'll give you a day or two to gather the necessary equipment and then we'll release Sharon."

We handed him a copy of Sharon's Living Will which we made out when she was first admitted to Magee. It was the living will, or the official declaration of what to do in the event that Sharon could no longer communicate what lengths hospital staff should take to keep her alive.

"No tubal feedings," Sharon shuddered. "And no ventilator," she waved an emphatic hand in front of her. We bent our heads together as Sharon finished looking over the form, making final decisions. She scrawled her signature and dated it, and I handed it back to Dr. Cartright, who discreetly left.

Signing the living will cast a pall over the room. Heavy-hearted, I held my head in my hands for a moment. Then I lifted it up, suddenly forgetting myself. She had closed her eyes and seemed to have drifted off.

I reached over and petted her hand. "Babe?"

"I'm here, sweetheart." Her eyelids shuttered her emotions.

"So it all boils down to this? Seven years of fighting to stand up to this damn cancer and ..."

"Our life is in God's hands every day," she said. "Sick or well, we all have a time." She wet her lips. Her words came out very slowly as if she didn't want to waste precious breaths. "I want to go ... and be with you ... in our lovely home, ... see my plants, ... feel breezes ... *real* sunshine ... stream in ... through the window."

"You love summertime." I looked around. This room held no color. It offered nothing in the way of hope that Shar needed to lift her spirits. She would be merely existing here. Of course, she needed to be home.

I studied her hands. *Thank God, the edema is gone.* I took one hand into mine and held it, gently caressing her palm, her knuckles, each delicate finger. She had red, painful looking hangnails and the nail itself was cracked.

Does the air in here cause that? When I rubbed my thumb over them, they felt hot and brittle. Her skin looked translucent. I buried my face in her chest for a moment. I could hear her heartbeat through the thin, cotton hospital gown. She smelled of antiseptic soap and menthol ointment.

I recalled other fragrances—like Shalimar and Destiny, Shar's signature perfumes—recognized from years of living with her. She'd daub the scent behind each ear lobe and drip a few drops to the front of her blouse—an enchanting vapor that clung to the soft cloth. Those beautiful, carefree moments of our life together were dissipating like a morning mist. We couldn't stop it from happening.

The sounds came from deep inside of me, deep sobs I couldn't stop. Wracked with such unmanly emotion, I tried to stand up and move away so I wouldn't frighten her or—

heaven forbid—make her even sadder. But oh God, this

fragile woman I'd given my heart to fourteen years earlier

held me to her side with one hand firmly over mine and

spoke softly, "Shhhh, we'll take it day-by-day." She sang,

"*I got you, babe…*"

The fact she was carrying a tune in her condition

surprised the hell out of me.

I sang back, *"…Babe" For some reason I could*

remember all of the words, but I would loudly sing, "I Got

You Babe."

We could always blend our voices together, but the

grief we felt made it sound even better as we finished the

refrain. "I Got You Babe."

My voice cracked and disappeared altogether a couple

of times when I tried to sing the next stanza about the

flowers in the spring and how I got her to wear my wedding

ring. *Now that's a story.*

"You proposed … on the day … of our golf course … adventure." She outlined my jaw lightly with her fingertips.

"What took me so long?"

She closed her eyes and seemed to search her mind for the words. Then she sang the part about when she was sad, I was her clown, and if she got scared, I was always around —it came out more of a cross between singing and speaking.

This got me where she lived…"In my heart.." I'd made that a priority. She would never have to go through anything alone. A jarring truth hit me—the perfect *timing* of our relationship. God had freed me up when I retired. Before that, I was so damn busy. But after Sharon's cancer came, God removed the obstacles.

I told Sharon about my epiphany.

"Thank you, Father," she said softly. The light blanket was balled up at the far end of the bed and her sheet hung over the edge. I knelt down next to her and arranged them as I tried to pull myself together. In the process, we ended up holding each other and crying together.

Sometime later, I don't remember how long, I picked up the thread of the Sonny and Cher song—the same one that was playing when we walked hand-in-hand after our wedding vows.

I felt like I was back in the church again when I told her to put her little hand in mind, that there wasn't any hill or mountain we couldn't climb. The lyrics seemed sacred, and we both knew we'd been living them out.

I looked into my wife's eyes. Deep green eyes stared back, full of love. As we sang the end of the song to each other, my heart somehow felt lighter. She had a goofy grin on her face. Our circumstances hadn't changed, but our mood had improved.

I looked at my watch. If I wanted Shar home, I'd have to check into the health care equipment I'd need. I consulted the list Dr. Cartright left with us and checked off a few more items and circled the phone number for Hospice.

"Honey, I need to get these things for the house. We're going to bust you out of here as soon as I can."

"Go get 'em," she whispered.

***

I pulled into the driveway, and wheeled Sharon into the house.

"Joe, help me stand." She sighed with pleasure, as if to say *I'm really home.* I'd put some of her small plants and a few fragrant candles around the room to welcome her back.

She leaned on me as we stepped into the living room, taking them in. Her gaze went to the framed photographs of us on one end table and several pictures of her sons on the other. She sought out her paintings, lingering for a moment on the one we called *Beginnings.* Her eyes trailed the furniture and back to me. "Aaaahh," she breathed. Her eyes misted up and she brought her hands to her heart. "How I've waited for this day," she said in a trembling voice.

"Welcome home," I whispered, taken by her emotion.

"You have no idea how happy I am."

I squeezed her hand. "Your face tells it all."

"I see you got the equipment…" Her voice faltered.

"*Voila.* Your new bed," I said, pointing to an electrically-powered bed in the living room. "We can raise it during the day so you can watch your birds and admire the plants outside, the ones you picked out for the front yard," I said, trying to make the view sound as inviting as possible. "We can lower it whenever you want to sleep, or if you're too uncomfortable to sit up."

I will so miss sleeping next to you...

I pointed to the bed. "Would you rather sit ... or lie down?"

"I'm a little tired." Just the little she said caused her to be out of breath.

I glanced at the silent oxygen machine stored in the corner of the living room. "Honey, do you think we should connect you up to the oxygen?"

She nodded. I loosened the sheets and blanket and laid her down on her back. Fluffing up the pillow, I placed it behind her back, then adjusted the angle of her bed. "Comfortable?"

She gave a slight nod.

I glimpsed a movement out of the corner of my eye.

"Look Shar, there's a robin on the windowsill." *If only it were a cardinal or more exotic bird to welcome her. But a robin will do.*

I unwound the twenty or so feet of tubing attached to the oxygen machine and hooked Sharon up to the cannula. I switched it on, and a loud hum filled the air.

"Thank you, honey," she said with a contented smile and drifted off to sleep.

When Sharon woke up, she looked around the room. She seemed to be searching for something. "What do you want, Shar? Something to eat? A glass of water? Are you in pain? What are you looking for?"

She looked away from me as she muttered, "Toilet."

I wondered if I should take her to our bathroom or start out with the ugly but utilitarian Port-a-John now adorning our living room. Eight square feet of plastic sheeting lay under the toilet to protect the carpet. I set down the Sudoku puzzle I was filling out on the end table. *Might as well use the port-a-john.* I pulled the living room curtains shut and turned on the light in the corner. *Okay, now the toilet.* I picked it up and set it down closer to the bed. *Time to get Sharon.* Leaning over the bed, I positioned Sharon's arms around my neck and scooped her frail body into my arms. She didn't weigh much. Three or four baby steps later, we made it to the commode and I helped her sit down. "You okay?"

"Yes." She fixed her eyes on the wall and avoided my gaze.

Uh-oh. She needs privacy. I disappeared into the kitchen around the corner. There, I puttered about rearranging, cleaning, and waiting for Sharon to call me.

"Jooooeee?"

At the sound of her voice, I returned the living room. I first went to her bed, rearranging the bed covers. Then I went to Sharon, lifted her in my arms, and carried her back to the freshly-made bed.

"Shar, are you hungry?"

She considered. "I could eat a little something."

"How about a soft-boiled egg? I've also made some cherry jello. Does that sound good? And I have a high-protein shake the doctors recommended to keep up your strength. I tasted it. It's not bad at all. At least it'll give you something to wash your food down with."

"Sure."

I scooted over a new utility tray table on wheels purchased just for her meals. I carried in the cooked egg and her protein shake, set them down and raised the tray so Shar could reach the food. The gelatin jiggled in its small bowl when I set it down.

That night I couldn't bear to sleep in our bed. In fact, I wondered if I'd ever be able to do so again. A restless movement from Shar interrupted my thoughts. *Does she feel how odd our situation is now, or is she beyond that?*

She motioned me to come closer. "Joe, don't leave. Stay near me."

"I'm right here." Pulling the recliner next to the bed, I took her hand. "I'm not going anywhere."

As I sat there listening, unfamiliar sounds—the incessant humming of the machine transporting oxygen to my wife, and the creak of her bed as she turned over, a slight moan, some sighs—mixed with the familiar—the ticking of the grandfather clock and the sound of the air conditioner starting up a new cycle—all of these sounds mingling in the semi-dark room. Everything seemed unnaturally loud. I glanced at Sharon who would jerk involuntarily from time to time. I put on some soft piano music in hopes that it would soothe and carry her off to sleep.

Somewhere in the dark hours of that night, maybe before dawn broke, truth began to creep into my consciousness. *This will be the last bed Shar sleeps in. That'll make it her…*I refused to let the word into my mind. But I couldn't ignore what I now understood, what Shar had already come to terms with. I couldn't escape reality. My bargaining days with God had finally ended.

How long do we have? Will it happen quickly? Or will it be drawn out, with Shar in pain? Lord, I don't want her to suffer. How will we cope at the end?

Early the next morning, I leaned over Shar's sleeping form. *Good morning, Sunshine.* She must have felt my breath as I checked on her because she opened her eyes. Shar was never an early riser. "Honey, go back to sleep," I whispered. But she needed to go to the bathroom.

The day had begun

We soon established a familiar routine. After a light

breakfast, we'd read the Bible together and discuss various passages, exploring how they applied to our lives. We'd stop, and I'd do some housework. After adjusting her bed to a more upright position, Shar would look out the window and admire the view. I'd put on some music for her. She'd often get a visitor. Whether we stayed alone or company came, she loved to knit. When she had a guest, they'd sit and talk. I'd wander in and out of the room, watering the plants or offering cups of hot or iced tea along with custard or gelatin so Shar could eat, too.

One morning, right on schedule, the doorbell rang. I swung the door open and saw the familiar Hospice van at the curb. But on the top step stood a new woman carrying a bulky plastic bag. She held out her hand and said cheerfully, "Hi Mr. Belan. You don't know me. I'm Stephanie, the new girl on the block. I've come to give your, um, wife, a bath."

"Come on in." I turned and said a little louder, "Shar, it's time for your bath."

Stephanie lowered the bed and gave her a sponge bath. As they bonded, I could hear light chatter and lots of laughter as I listened from from my spot in the kitchen. "You girls okay in there? I hear an awful lot of splashing going on," I teased. They laughed since 'splashing' was impossible at this point.

"Just fine, Mr. Belan," the Hospice employee called back.

After the sponge bath, the caretaker helped Sharon get back into bed and adjusted it to a comfortable position so that she could sit up and chat. "I'm thinking you could use a little bit of pampering about now…" Stephanie pulled out a nail kit. "I give outstanding manicures."

My wife had never been interested in that kind of thing before but must have consented because when I peeked in,

I saw the woman had set a flat board across Shar's lap. Stephanie got started right away. The smell of hand lotion filled the air as she gently massaged my wife's hands.

"That feels so good," Shar exclaimed. "The color's pretty, like pink pearls."

When Stephanie finished, she said, "Mr. Belan—"

"My name's Joe," I called from the kitchen.

"Joe, come see your wife's beautiful manicure."

"Honey, my nails shimmer…" Sharon waved them in the air at me. She giggled like a teenager.

As Shar grew weaker, we'd simplified our lifestyle to the bare minimum. I stopped cooking. Neighbors and people from the church brought in meals, which helped a lot. I left briefly and only if someone came to stay with Sharon. Otherwise, I stayed close to her so we could be together. I'd remind her of things we'd done in our travels or when we were dating. She loved to hear the details.

We spent hours rating the Steelers' current line-up, still at camp in pre-season scrimmages. It was such a disappointment to both of us that Shar couldn't make many of the games the year before. We'd attended thirteen straight seasons of the Steelers' games. I had to be thankful.

I realized yet again that Shar was not only my wife, she was my best friend.

One afternoon as I finished folding a set of sheets, towels and washcloths, I looked up to see Sharon watching. "I thought you were asleep," I said stacking the pieces by size.

"God gave me the best caregiver in the world," she said. Her green eyes softened as she tried to show me her gratitude. "Funny … caring … hard-working…"

"God knew what He was doing when He put us together," I said, my voice catching. "You are my inspiration."

As Shar's immune system continued to falter, the bad days grew more frequent. A number of changes occurred. She ate little and couldn't sit up very much. She also had sudden coughing fits—so many that Hospice brought a contraption called a nebulizer to the house to ease her breathing. I dangled it in my hands and looked it at it from several angles. With a little imagination, I decided the part of the apparatus Shar had to breathe through looked a little like a pipe. I envisioned us in the midst of a Native American scene—some kind of tribal pow-wow. Immediately after, we'd seat ourselves around a big fire and negotiate.

"We make peace," I said holding up the nebulizer so Sharon could see it and scraped some kind of medicine into the nebulizer cup. I connected one end of the tubing to the machine and plugged it into the wall. I connected the other end of the tubing into a shorter, wider clear "pipe" specially designed to inhale the medicine. It would go directly to her lungs when she breathed.

"You. Mouth. Breathe." When she did, short puffs of air emerged. "Me want peace pipe now," I demanded, holding out my hand. I pretended to smoke it.

She coughed. "More peace pipe. Me," she said, entering into the game.

We passed it back and forth a few turns until I gave it to her for good. "Me. You. Friends now."

As the medicine finished, she handed the nebulizer back to me. "You. Very good chief." She'd stopped coughing for the moment.

"Joe, potty time."

As uncouth as it might sound, I enjoyed the closeness that we shared during those bathroom breaks. We'd go through the rituals of closing the drapes, turning on the light with me carrying her to the toilet. The one thing that changed with Sharon is that she ceased to be embarrassed about accidents. As the cancer progressed, she'd have one or two accidents a day. But it didn't matter to either of us anymore. The barriers disappeared. Sometimes just the effort of getting out of bed, or back into bed would cause Sharon to have an accident. I always placed a large, soft pad on the bed in order to absorb any spills if this happened.

Up until the very end, Shar maintained a modicum of modesty on the toilet. Even then, I knew she wanted privacy. So I took that time to remove and replace the soiled bed pad, sheets, blankets, towels and nightgown. Making sure that Sharon had everything within reaching distance, I took everything to the basement, rinsed them out and threw them into the washing machine. With that task out of the way, I'd return to Sharon. When she was unable to do it herself, I cleaned her most private parts.

When I picked her up and lowered her onto the bed again, I would maintain my hold on her in a prolonged hug until she said, "Enough." She knew what I was doing and smiled lovingly, touching my face as if to memorize it with her fingers while I moved away from her.

Then I tenderly washed and dried her bottom, then applied medicated salve before covering her with an adult diaper and a clean nightgown. I'd finish by pulling up the sheet and adjusting her pillow.

On Shar's worst days, I wracked my brain to recollect funny incidents to entertain her. As she swallowed her pain, I tried to make her as comfortable as possible. Then I sat down next to her and brought up one of our stories or a funny incident.

On one such day, I was too tired and sad to think clearly. But as I looked around the room, I saw the candles I'd placed there to make it smell nice. Two rose-scented and two violet-scented ones. I suddenly had an inspiration.

"Do you remember Nurse Ratched? At Magee?"

She coughed. I thought I saw the ends of her mouth turn up.

"I stood up and admonished in a loud, brassy voice, "There will be no lighting of candles in this room, sir. It's an oxygen hazard." I put my hands on my hips and strutted over to the vanilla candle and with two fingers, pretended to snuff it out. I shook my breasts and went to another candle. I turned to Sharon and made my crabbiest face. "No candles means NO candles."

She held out a weak hand to me. As I took it in my own, I heard a barely audible, "Thanks."

I was losing her more each day. I would tell her the stories, not only to make her smile, but to bridge the gap that was widening between us each day—the one between life and death.

It scared me.

September 24, 2009, I sat in the living room with members of my wife's family. I could hear the hum of the oxygen machine and Sharon's slow breathing—but not much else. Reverend Palmer was chatting to me, but I had no idea what he was saying.

I had the weird sense that Sharon was looking directly into my soul for a moment. I turned and mouthed the words, "I love you" to her. And I think I saw a gentle acknowledging nod in return. Her eyes then went blank.

Stuart choked out, "Joe, she's, God, my mom's ...." He could not make himself say the words.

All eyes were on me as I rose and moved to her side, once again hugging her and burying my face in the pillow next to her head. I kissed her lips, eyes, forehead, and what little hair she still had. Holding her hands I couldn't help but think about how fast her hands grew cold.

The intense silence caught me off guard. I had to fill it. I had to say something.

"Shar, I will love you forever. You are in God's hands in death just as you were in life." Brave words for me, considering my world, as I knew it, had ceased to exist.

I wish that I could tell you the time she died. It was not significant then—and even if I look on the death certificate now, it's only a series of numbers. I'm sure that it was late afternoon or early evening. Someone called the Great Lakes Hospice people. It might have been me. Upon their arrival, everything moved ahead at warp speed and together we prepared her to be moved to the funeral home. With family gathered around her, the Reverend said a prayer.

The house would never feel like a home again.

Chapter 17
THE FUNERAL

I kicked into hyper-organization mode as I addressed the family a few hours later. "This is the deal. Today's Sunday. *Still?* I've called the funeral home. I got a bag of Sharon's belongings together. Her sister Paula found the gown Sharon wore at Matt's wedding. We bagged up her favorite wig and some of her toiletries. I've boxed up the gold cross necklace she always wore along with her engagement and wedding rings. I'll include some photos in the bag so the mortician will have a better idea of how to make her up. I'm going to drop them off at the funeral home tomorrow morning."

Paula looked at me. "Which one?"

"Dusckas, on Sterretania Road."

I continued. "We'll hold the viewing from Wednesday

to Friday. Sharon had a lot of friends. I'm guessing we'll need that extra day to accommodate the many who will want to pay their respects."

Everyone seemed fine with these plans. I turned to the Reverend. "Lou, I'd like to have the service on Saturday morning. Can you accommodate us?"

"Certainly." He double-checked her date of birth and a few other pertinent facts but had the rest mapped out in his mind. "She discussed the key scriptures she wanted me to preach on. That makes it easier. Always helps when a person is as organized as your wife was." *I thought, "Yeah, right. Sharon was the least organized person that I knew."*

Always has been that way. I briefly recalled the detailed lesson plans for the substitute she always made prior to missing any time in the classroom. She would work on those plans for hours.

"Yes." I cleared my throat. "She even planned her own

eulogy, which Gregg will read after your talk."

The Reverend looked confused. "And … Gregg is?"

"Sharon's brother-in-law," I said, with a sweep of my arm.

Gregg nodded. "That's me. I've got it right here."

I hesitated. "I'll make you a copy." Suddenly anxious to hold onto anything she wrote in her own hand, I coveted the original.

"After the service, we'll give the floor over to those who knew Sharon. They may want to tell a funny story or anecdote, or talk about her strength. Whatever." I paused, briefly reeling through happy memories as if they were motion pictures. *What did I want to share?* The family was silent. I suppose they were thinking of their own stories.

Stuart stood up and stretched. "Is there going to be any music?"

"Of course. Sharon pre-selected all the music to be

played and sung."

"That's cool."

"Any questions?" Everyone seemed clear on what would happen. As the family meeting broke up, the bell rang. I walked over to the door.

A tall thin man with a trim beard and moustache held out his hand. "I'm Ed Harvey, from Great Lakes Hospice. My condolences to the family," he said quietly including everyone in his kind gaze. "Which one of you is Mr. Belan?"

"I am. Call me Joe." I shook his hand, noticing he had a surprisingly strong grip for such a lean fellow.

"I'm here to take the deceased to the funeral home," he stated quietly. He spoke with me for several minutes in the living room, then excused himself. When he returned, he was carrying a gurney and what looked like some professionally-laundered sheets. He set them down on top of it. Ed looked up. "Has everyone in the family said goodbye to the deceased?"

"Yes, yes, they have."

He laid a hand on my shoulder. "Joe, you might want to the call the family together. They can watch if they'd like. Some feel more closure when they witness this leave-taking. Others want to keep a wide berth."

I rounded them up to the living room. Her immediate family huddled together and spoke in whispers. I stood close to Sharon, one hand on the bedrail. The Reverend stood nearby, his arms in front and hands folded. His presence brought calm to the room, and I was grateful he'd chosen to be here with us at this critical time. Good man, that Lou. Not only a man of the cloth and devotion to God, but over the years, he'd been a personal friend to Sharon and me.

Ed took the floor. "I know this is difficult for you. I

won't need any of your assistance, so feel free to take a seat if that will make you feel more comfortable. I'm going to place this sheet on the gurney." He unfolded a king-sized creased sheet and centered it on the gurney so that the edge hung just above the floor. "It's all natural fiber," he said, as if assuring us that Shar would have a high-quality shroud of sorts.

I watched Ed as he brought the gurney closer to the bed.

"I'm just going to remove her from the bed and place her on the gurney."

"Can I help y—" I asked. *Force of habit, I guess.*

"No, no, no, no. Do not help me." Ed quickly countered. I got the feeling his response was a liability issue and backed off.

In the silence of the room, we watched him fold the sheet over Sharon's body in a few deft, practiced steps. The last thing he did was to pull the sheet over her head. I flinched in spite of myself.

"Now I'm going to strap the body to the gurney," he gently explained so we would all know what to expect. He tightened three white straps to secure her. "If someone can just hold the door," he instructed.

Stuart got it. I alone followed Ed to his vehicle. Wordlessly, I opened the hatchback door for him and watched him slide the gurney in. In a lightning-quick moment, I saw myself with Sharon as attendants closed the ambulance door the morning she rode to Magee.

I shivered. Shook my head to clear it. *God, I need a cigarette.* I hadn't smoked in years.

Ed closed the door with my beloved Sharon inside. As I watched him drive away, I had the strangest feeling. *She wasn't there.* Wasn't afraid anymore. Wouldn't be riding backwards in any more ambulances. Wouldn't be getting nauseated or dizzy. Sharon had no more hospitals to visit.

"Anyone want more coffee?" I asked, holding a lukewarm pot in my hand. "I have cold cuts here for sandwiches. The bread's on the counter. Help yourself. Condiments are on the top shelf of the fridge."

As the family sought comfort in food, Lou took me aside and sat me down on the couch. "Joe, how you holding up? A mighty tough day for you, I can tell."

I let out a long sigh, and with eyes closed, just nodded.

When the talk shifted to Sharon, he gently brought up a conversation they had before she passed away. In a daze, the sound of Lou's voice kept me seated more than anything he actually said. "You know, your wife was very concerned that with her passing, it might be too much for you to give a eulogy at the funeral."

"What do you mean?"

He leaned over and gave my shoulder a pat. "She

didn't want to make her passing any harder for you, Joe."

I shrugged. "How hard is it to give a speech? I gave talks to my students for years."

"Yeah, it's one thing to prepare an academic lecture. But quite another have to prepare something after losing your wife and soul-mate."

"You do what you have to do, Lou."

"Well, that may be. You'll have to make that decision. She said after all you went through with her, for once, she wanted others to think of you and meet your needs. She yearned for you to be consoled, not the consoler."

I closed my eyes and sank back on the sofa. Lou knew what a toll this had taken on me.

His compassionate eyes sought mine. "Up 'til now, you've done everything she's wanted you to do. Why don't you consider honoring this last wish? Do you think you could do that? She loved you so much."

"I know. I'll give it some thought."

"That's all I'm saying, Joe. That's all you need to do. I'm here for you, brother. The whole congregation is. Shall we have a word of prayer before I return you to your family?"

As Lou prayed, I bowed my head and imagined Shar seated next to God, pointing down at me. "That's my husband, Joe," she'd say. "Be extra kind to him tonight."

After everyone had cleared out of the house, I collapsed into the recliner in the living room. With the oxygen machine switched off, the silence turned eerie. I got up and walked through the empty rooms of the house. Every room had a memory. I backed out of the bedroom. I tried to block out the times we'd danced around the house to real music or songs inside my head. The times we made love afterward.

Do something constructive. Get to work.

I stripped the sheets off the hospital bed and took them downstairs to put into into the washer for the last time. As I waited for them to go through the wash cycle, I sanitized the toilet bucket for the last time. The buzzer sounded and I tossed the sheets into the dryer. I went into the kitchen and washed the coffee pot along with the few cups and saucers we'd used earlier. *It's probably time to take the bed sheets out now.* I liked the feel of the hot sheets as I folded them up into large tidy squares. I lay them on the end of Shar's stripped down hospital bed. They were ready for pick-up.

With nothing else left to do, I stood in the middle of the living room near the bed, the place that Sharon had occupied the major part of the past month and a half. Our small world had revolved around it. I stood fifteen, maybe twenty minutes before I sank to the floor on my knees. *Oh, God. Sharon. Sharon!* I'd kept myself under check since *it* happened and did the tasks at hand. But now, alone in this empty house, the hot, slow tears come. I didn't try to hold back anymore. Suddenly, it didn't matter. I had no one to be strong for.

Sharon is gone. This set me off. Racked with tears, my shoulders heaved as I cried. *I want to hold you again. Just wrap my arms around you. I want you. I want you. Sharon!*

I rocked back and forth, my head in my hands as I wept. I don't know how long I knelt there on the carpet keening for the loss of the one love that could never be replaced. I grasped at torn and frayed tissues sodden with nose drippings and tears. Slowly the fading light outside the window turned to full darkness. My leg muscles cramped. My joints ached. My knees felt like they'd give out. I turned and sat.

I thought about her funeral and I wondered how I'd ever be able to put into words what she meant to me. Thinking of that task overwhelmed me.

Right again, Shar. I can't even think beyond this moment, let alone talk about how happy you made me. I half-laughed and half-cried. *Shar, you knew me better than I did myself. You always wanted to protect me. We always did that for each other.*

I must have wandered into the recliner at some point. I woke up in the middle of the night still aching with the raw need to hold my wife. I spied the half-finished afghan Shar had been knitting for the past month or so and took it from the back of the sofa. I touched the soft yarn, brought it to my nose and inhaled. The green and brown threads smelled of her sweetness. I closed my eyes and recalled the way the yarn slid through her fingers, the deftness of her movements—until she lost the ability to manipulate the needles. In my mind's eye, I saw her smooth and stretch out the piece after she finished a row. She'd look at me. Not bad. These threads were one of the last things she'd touched. *How is it possible for this small, unfinished patch of yarn to connect me to her?* I closed my eyes and laid it over me. My arms and legs stuck out from beneath it, but I felt comforted at last.

When I woke up next, it was six a.m.

Out of habit, my gaze went straight to the hospital bed. *Empty.* No smile or even a blink. *The sooner I get that bed out of here, the better.*

I prepared myself a light breakfast. After tidying up, I made a list of the people I needed to call and errands I had to get done today. I put Hospice at the top of the list. Even though I was busy preparing for the viewing, the days seemed to crawl by.

***

Wednesday finally arrived. At the funeral home, we

placed the last painting Shar had done next to the casket. We'd called it "Beginnings" because it depicted a new day. Typical of all her work, the canvas included a conglomeration of scenes taken from several landscapes. It had the right mix of clouds with the morning sun's rays peeking through them and shining onto some several tall, thin pine trees in the mist. In the foreground she'd painted the tops of some weeds poking up through the marsh. I stared at it now. She was off on 'Another Excellent Sharon Adventure.' *This time without Joe.*

My mom looked over and held out an arm to steady me. "You okay, Joe?"

I took a shaky breath. "Yes, I'm fine."

The mortician did a good job on my wife. Except for looking waxy and thin, her make-up flattered her. People remarked about how good she looked for all she'd gone through. After one of these comments, I had a déjà vu. The time that Shar's ex came to the same funeral we did. I told

Shar, "You look more stunning than the deceased." Now it

came back to haunt me.

There was a tremendous outpouring of love and

support from family and friends, colleagues and neighbors.

A steady stream of people filled the funeral home each day.

At times, it seemed the line of people would never end. It

was very tiring to repeat the same story over and over.

Though after a while, I felt like a robot, but I was still very

grateful for their presence. Between viewings, our entire

family went to my house to rest, eat and recharge. Some

days I didn't say anything the entire time. Other days I

couldn't stop talking. I didn't have to explain myself.

Family, it seems always understands.

One afternoon when we returned, my sister pointed out

yet another arrangement of flowers "Look at the roses," she

exclaimed. She read the heartfelt message attached. "It's

from the team at MD Anderson."

"Really?" I made sure to send them a copy of her obituary the day it came out. The card stock had a colored rainbow on it. I smiled. Little touches like that made a difference. Sharon would've loved it.

We left the funeral home after a heartfelt service where many people spoke of how Shar inspired them with her courage and optimism. I talked about the organ music we'd had over the three days. "They were happy songs, and Shar wanted you to be happy." *Just a few words, Shar, don't worry. I'm so glad I added that extra day. Did you see how many people loved you?*

Saturday morning found us at the church for the service. Lou came right over and took me into a bear hug. "We're here for you, brother. You will get through this with the family of God."

Following the service, we headed to Laurel Hill

Cemetery and her interment. Afterward, I slipped off by myself. I looked up and to my amazement, didn't see a single cloud. Just bright sunshine and blue sky. A perfect golf day for me. Exactly like the day I received that fateful phone call from Sharon when she had her physical and our life changed.

I had the oddest feeling she'd gathered all the clouds together and moved them out of the way so that nothing would obstruct her view. She was now shining straight down on me. *It's a sign from her.* "Good morning, Sunshine," I whispered.

EPILOGUE

Two years later I rose early in the morning with plans to go to the cemetery. Outside the window, the leaves swirled down, marking yet another year of your passing. I decided to wear a thick, tan cable-knit sweater—a final birthday gift from Shar—and one I hardly ever wore. I gently tugged it out of the drawer and slipped it over my head. As I pulled my arms through, a folded piece of white paper dropped onto the floor from the right sleeve.

It lay where it landed as I stared. Then it registered. Could it be…? "You sneaky little stinker. You hid a note up the sleeve."

When did you do that? How did you get it there without me seeing? How many others are there around the house?

My heart beat faster as I bent to pick the paper. I held

it for a minute, speculating what beautiful words lay inside,

wanting to savor the wonder. Finally, I couldn't wait any

longer. I unfolded the paper.

> *My darling,*
> *I hope this keeps you warm all day!*
> *x o x o*
> *Love you forever!*
> *Sharon*

The paper smelled faintly of your Shalimar. I folded

your note and put it in my pocket. I felt as if you're right

here with me, and yes, I was feeling warm today.

Ready to go.

I loaded the back of my Ford Explorer with a flat of

impatiens I bought for you, some mulch and a spade along

with everything else to spruce up your gravesite. I've got

my lawn chair and a new James Patterson novel to read

after I finish planting the flowers. Did I remember to bring

it all? I know. You used to make fun of me for writing

everything down. But lists are good things. I've got mine right here.

After you left this world, I had a lot of bad days. Once in awhile I miss you so much I can't even get out of bed. But today's a good day, Shar. Especially now that I found your note. Plus, I'm wearing the sweater you bought for me. I can't believe you left me another note. You always make me smile.

I turned into the driveway of Laurel Hill Cemetery and pulled up next to Sharon's grave. "Those jerks!" I cursed under my breath at how the workers had such a wanton disregard for the gravesites. "They've weed-whacked over your flowers and left the weeds again." I told the cemetery administrator about it, but he couldn't seem to stop it from happening. I swore. *Oh, sorry, Shar. I did it again. I know how you frown on that kind of language. Remind God that I'm really a good guy and I'm trying to clean up my act.*

Maybe, with your help we can convince Him to let me be with you.

As I talked, I knelt and pulled the creeping ground clover and errant crabgrass that encroached on her flower bed. I planted the red impatiens. I'd always liked these hardy flowers because they bloomed well into the first frost. With the last plant in and mulched, I sat down and rested.

I wondered what other visitors thought of Sharon's grave. I wanted them to be able to say, "Someone is buried here who was greatly loved." I stood up and looked at the gravesite. Sharon would be pleased.

Perspiration trickled down the back of my neck. "It's warrn for September, Shar."

I suddenly felt a refreshing breeze blow across my face and down my collar. But when I looked up, the few trees around me were motionless. I didn't see any leaves rustling or a single branch swaying. Nothing was moving. Not a blade of grass. Not a ripple in any of the flags on the gravestones. Strange. Where had that breeze come from?

I shook my head to clear it and sat down in my lawn chair to read my book.

I felt the breeze again, this time distinctly ruffling my hair. The pages of the book blew back to Chapter One. I looked around and, again, found my surroundings undisturbed, motionless. "What the heck…?"

The sun came out and shone across the page of my book and over my hand. Bright beautiful sunshine. Again, weird. It had been hazy, not sunny at all. I shaded my eyes with my hand and looked up at the sky. Rays of bright, beautiful sunshine came out from behind the clouds.

My skin prickled. Goosebumps appeared on my arms. Many people think when something like this happens, it's a loved one sending a message to them. Is it that … or is it simply a breeze and a dose of my overactive imagination? But how do I account for the sunshine?

Is it you, Sharon? Will I always wonder when something like this happens? How can I tell if it's something ordinary or some kind of supernatural force or a message from you?

I looked up in the sky as if I actually expected her to answer my questions. "Shar, am I totally insane here? Or are you here with me? Is this a sign from you?"

The sunshine steadily poured down on me—is that an answer? Oh my God, Sharon.

I haven't lost you.

"Shar, you aren't here in the ground." I pointed to the sky. "You are there." I pointed to the trees. "You are there." I pointed to the clouds. "You are there."

Then I touched my heart and said, "And—you are here. *Always.*"